ATHEROSCLEROSIS REVIEWS
Volume 21

Prevention and Noninvasive Therapy
of Atherosclerosis

Atherosclerosis Reviews

Chief Editors: Antonio M. Gotto and Rodolfo Paoletti

Atherosclerosis Reviews
Volume 21

Prevention and Noninvasive Therapy of Atherosclerosis

Editors

Alexander Leaf, M.D.
Departments of Medicine and
* Preventive Medicine*
Harvard Medical School
Massachusetts General Hospital
Boston, Massachusetts

Peter C. Weber, M.D.
Universität München
Institut für Prophylaxe und
* Epidemiologie der Kreislaufkrankheiten*
München, F.R.G.

Raven Press New York

Raven Press, 1185 Avenue of the Americas, New York, New York 10036

Made in the United States of America

Library of Congress Cataloging-in-Publication Data

Prevention and noninvasive therapy of atherosclerosis / editors,
    Alexander Leaf. Peter C. Weber.
        p. cm.—(Atherosclerosis reviews: v. 21)
      Presentations from the International Workshop on Atherosclerosis:
Prevention and Noninvasive Therapy, which took place in Key West
from Nov. 30 till Dec. 2, 1989.
      Includes bibliographical references.
      ISBN 0-88167-685-3 (v. 1).
      1. Atherosclerosis—Prevention—Congresses. 2. Atherosclerosis—
Congresses. I. Leaf, Alexander, 1920– . II. Weber, Peter C.
III. International Workshop on Atherosclerosis: Prevention and
Noninvasive Therapy (1989: Key West, Fla.) IV. Series.
     [DNLM: 1. Arteriosclerosis—prevention & control—congresses.
2. Arteriosclerosis—therapy—congresses. W1 AT385 v. 21 / WG 550
P944 1989]
RC692.A729 vol. 21
616.1'36 s—dc20
[616.1'36]
DNLM/DLC
for Library of Congress   90-8445
                                               CIP

9 8 7 6 5 4 3 2

Acknowledgments

On behalf of all participants in the International Workshop on Atherosclerosis: Prevention and Noninvasive Therapy, which took place in Key West from November 30 until December 2, 1989, we thank BAYER AG for making the workshop possible. We are especially grateful to Dr. Jürgen Fritsch, Mr. Klaus Gerressen, Dr. Klaus-Jürgen Preuß, and Dr. Günther Thomas for their invaluable contribution to the success of the Workshop.

Contents

Foreword

Doctors Leaf and Weber have produced an exemplary series of papers that provide a comprehensive review of atherosclerosis and its clinical complications. The review spans the breadth of biomedical science from molecular and cellular biological aspects of the vessel wall to epidemiologic data and clinical trials. The topics covered in this review are quite varied, but they all relate to a theme of prevention and noninvasive therapy.

This volume of *Atherosclerosis Reviews* represents a wealth of material for the student of atherosclerosis. The conclusions and summaries present a fascinating perspective from a diverse group of authors. Many of the unresolved questions and unexplained confounding results in the field of atherosclerosis and coronary heart disease (CHD) are described. For example, the original populations of the Seven Countries Study and of the Framingham Study are now reaching advanced ages, and the latest epidemiologic data suggest that the pattern of risk factor relationship to CHD is seen to change over time and with age. Thus, intervention trials in the future must take into account these shifts in baseline population characteristics.

Antonio M. Gotto, Jr., M.D.
Rodolfo Paoletti, M.D.

Preface

This book contains the presentations at the first Bayer AG "International Workshop on Atherosclerosis," held in Key West, Florida on November 31–December 2, 1989.

The contents cover broad and important areas of both clinical and research understanding of atherosclerosis. These include the epidemiology, pathogenesis, and prevention of and noninvasive therapies for atherosclerosis. Experts in these areas have reviewed the present status of knowledge in these areas. With research moving as rapidly on all fronts as it is with atherosclerosis, it is important that the various views of the disease be seen together. What epidemiologic studies first taught us has now been tested through clinical trials. These, in turn, have stimulated laboratory studies that are clarifying the details of the atherosclerotic process at the cellular and molecular levels.

As atherogenesis is better understood, new facts will undoubtedly lead to preventive and therapeutic interventions that affect the atherosclerotic process more directly than do current approaches. Much attention today is given to the role of cholesterol in atherosclerosis. As important as cholesterol is, it is becoming evident that changes in the arterial wall must occur before low-density lipoprotein (LDL) cholesterol has a site to deposit. The nature of these early lesions and the factors involved in their development and growth into mature obstructing atheroma are being elucidated. As the details are filled in, we can anticipate multiple sites that will serve as potential targets for therapeutic and preventive interventions. Factors that affect platelet activity and the clotting mechanisms in blood and vessel wall, such as aspirin, are examples of such interventions.

These are exciting times in the understanding of atherosclerosis, the leading cause of death and a major cause of morbidity in all Western industrialized countries. It is the aim of this, the first Bayer AG "International Workshop on Atherosclerosis," and subsequent workshops to provide an overview of the progress in atherosclerosis research. We hope that the workshops will improve communication between investigators studying atherosclerosis from their respective disciplinary approaches—epidemiologic, clinical, morphological, biochemical, molecular, and genetic. We hope that this volume also serves a similar useful function for a broader audience.

Alexander Leaf, M.D.
Peter C. Weber, M.D.

Contributors

Keaven Anderson
Framingham Heart Study
5 Thurber Street
Framingham, Massachusetts 01701

Mari-Anna Berg
Department of Epidemiology
National Public Health Institute
Mannerheimintie 166
SF-00300 Helsinki, Finland

David H. Blankenhorn
Department of Medicine
Atherosclerosis Research Institute
University of Southern California School
of Medicine
2025 Zonal Avenue
Los Angeles, California 90033

Fritz R. Bühler
Department Forschung
Ordinariat Pathologie
Universitätskliniken
Kantonspital Basel
4031 Basel, Switzerland

Julie E. Buring
Departments of Medicine and Preventive
Medicine
Brigham and Women's Hospital
Harvard Medical School
55 Pond Avenue
Brookline, Massachusetts 02146

William Castelli
Framingham Heart Study
5 Thurber Street
Framingham, Massachusetts 01701

Agostino Faggiotto
Pharmacological Department
Bayer Italia S.p.A.
Via delle Groane, 126
20024 Garbaguate Milanese, Italy

Yuichiro Goto
Department of Medicine
Tokai University School of Medicine
Bohseidai, Isehara-shi
Kanagawa-ken 259-11, Japan

Jacek J. Hawiger
Department of Microbiology and
Immunology
Vanderbilt University School of
Medicine
Nashville, Tennessee 37232-2363

Charles H. Hennekens
Departments of Medicine and Preventive
Medicine
Brigham and Women's Hospital
Harvard Medical School
55 Pond Avenue
Brookline, Massachusetts 02146

E. Annie Higgs
The Wellcome Research Laboratories
Langley Court, Beckenham
Kent BR3 3BS, England

Ingvar Hjermann
Department of Medicine
Oslo University Medical School
Ullevaal Hospital
0407 Oslo 4, Norway

Leena Kartovaara
Department of Epidemiology
National Public Health Institute
Mannerheimintie 166
SF-00300 Helsinki, Finland

Ulrich Keil
Abt. f. Sozialmedizin und Epidemiologie
Ruhr Universität Bochum
Overbergstr. 17
4630 Bochum 1, F.R.G.

Ancel Keys
Department of Epidemiology
University of Minnesota
Stadium Gate 27
611 Beacon Street, S.E.
Minneapolis, Minnesota 55455

Heikki J. Korhonen
Department of Epidemiology
National Public Health Institute
Mannerheimintie 166
SF-00300 Helsinki, Finland

Alexander Leaf
Department of Medicine
Massachusetts General Hospital
Fruit Street
Boston, Massachusetts 02114

Paul Leren
Department of Medicine
Ullevaal Hospital
Medical Outpatient Clinic
0407 Oslo, Norway

Daniel Levy
Framingham Heart Study
5 Thurber Street
Framingham, Massachusetts 01701

Peter Libby
Tufts University School of Medicine
New England Medical Center
Cardiology Division
750 Washington Street
Boston, Massachusetts 02111

W. E. Miall
Sidegrath
Crook Road
Staveley, Kendal
Cumbria, LA8 9NN, England

Gero Miesenböck
Department of Medicine and Lipid
  Metabolism
University of Innsbruck
6020 Innsbruck, Austria

Salvador Moncada
The Wellcome Research Laboratories
Langley Court, Beckenham
Kent BR3 3BS, Kent, England

Emilio H. Moriguchi
Department of Medicine
Tokai University School of Medicine
Bohseidai, Isehara-shi
Kanagawa-ken 259-11, Japan

Aulikki Nissinen
University of Kuopio
Postbox 6
70211 Kuopio, Finland

Arne Nordoy
Department of Medicine
University of Tromso
9000 Tromso, Norway

Ralph S. Paffenbarger
Department of Epidemiology
Stanford University School of Medicine
Stanford, California 94305-5092

Richard M. J. Palmer
The Wellcome Research Laboratories
Langley Court, Beckenham
Kent BR3 3BS, England

Josef R. Patsch
Division of Clinical Atherosclerosis
Research
Department of Medicine
University of Innsbruck
6020 Innsbruck, Austria

Pirjo Pietinen
Department of Epidemiology
National Public Health Institute
Mannerheimintie 166
SF-00300 Helsinki, Finland

Pekka Puska
Department of Epidemiology
National Public Health Institute
Mannerheimintie 166
SF-003000 Helsinki, Finland

Russell Ross
Department of Pathology
University of Washington School of
Medicine
Health Science Building SM-30
Seattle, Washington 98195

Wolfgand Siess
Universität München
Institut für Prophylaxe und
Epidemiologie der
Kreislaufkrankheiten
Pettenkoferstr. 9
8000 München 2, F.R.G.

Jaakko Tuomilehto
Department of Epidemiology
National Public Health Institute
Mannerheimintie 166
SF-00300 Helsinki, Finland

Erkki Vartiainen
Department of Epidemiology
National Public Health Institute
Mannerheimintie 166
SF-00300 Helsinki, Finland

Peter C. Weber
Universität München
Institut für Prophylaxe und
Epidemiologie der
Kreislaufkrankheiten
Pettenkoferstrasse 9
8000 München 2, F.R.G.

Peter W. F. Wilson
Framingham Heart Study
5 Thurber Street
Framingham, Massachusetts 01701

Joseph L. Witztum
Department of Medicine, M013-D
University of California, San Diego
La Jolla, California 92093

Atherosclerosis Reviews, Volume 21,
edited by A. Leaf and P. C. Weber.
Raven Press, Ltd., New York © 1990.

Longevity, Coronary Disease, and Characteristics in Middle Age

Ancel Keys

Division of Epidemiology, School of Public Health, University of Minnesota,
Minneapolis, Minnesota

In epidemiological studies, we do not measure or see atherosclerosis; we only infer it from its product—coronary artery disease (CAD). Some pathologists have estimated the degree of coronary atherosclerosis and found no relation to body fatness. However, other variables were not evaluated and the samples used had questionable relevance, e.g., young soldiers killed in battle areas, patients dead from coronary artery disease compared with patients dead from other causes.

In 1946, newspaper accounts of coronary deaths of important executives brought to our attention a new problem. We wondered why some men were victims and others stayed well. What were the characteristics of those men that made some of them susceptible to coronary artery disease? We reasoned that recording the characteristics of healthy middle-aged executives and following them over the years would provide clues. So was born the Twin Cities Prospective Study (1).

The greatest concern with regard to coronary disease is its mortality and effect on longevity. I have emphasized longevity, as found in prospective studies of long duration. Discussed herein are the 40 years of follow-up in the Twin Cities Study (1), 24 years of study of men examined in Finland starting in 1956 (2), and 25 years of five cohorts in the Seven Countries Study (3,4). Coronary artery disease and characteristics found in relatively short-term studies may not be relevant to longevity.

THE 40-YEAR FOLLOW-UP OF MEN IN THE TWIN CITIES STUDY

The Minnesota subjects were executives aged 45 to 55 years at entry, representing 92% of the invited sample. They were given no advice at any time but the annual examination findings were sent to their personal physicians. In 40 years, 229 died, 90 from coronary artery disease, and 1 subject was lost to follow-up (Table 1). The first question is, How did the men who died differ at entry

1

TABLE 1. *Entry means: 64 alive and 219 dead after 40 years*

Measure	Alive	Dead	Alive minus dead
Body mass index	24.41	25.08	$t = -1.25$, $p = 0.21$
Mean skin folds	22.47	24.31	$t = -1.49$, $p = 0.14$
Relative girth	51.26	52.81	$t = -1.72$, $p = 0.09$
Body density	1.048	1.045	$t = 1.89$, $p = 0.06$

from the survivors? Several methods may be used to examine the relationship of mortality to entry characteristics. First is comparison of characteristics at entry of those who died with those of the survivors.

I will discuss body fat because the claim that it is an important risk factor has been questioned and reducing weight has become a billion-dollar business advertised for health as well as for cosmetic purposes.

Body fat was estimated by the body mass index (wt/ht^2), skin fold thickness (mm) over the triceps muscle, the tip of the scapula, and on the abdomen halfway between the umbilicus and the crest of the ilium, the abdominal girth divided by height, and the density of the body measured by underwater weighing adjusted for air in the respiratory system by nitrogen washout at the time of recording. There was no significant difference in any of four measures of fatness at entry between survivors and men who died from all causes or from coronary disease, but in the one-tailed comparison the CAD deaths had larger relative girth and lower body density. Those differences disappeared when allowance was made for blood pressure, which was correlated with all fatness measures, with $r = 0.3$ or more. They did not differ in either low- or high-density lipoprotein cholesterol or in smoking habits at entry. Almost all of the smokers had stopped long before death. Among 60 other entry characteristics, the only significant differences were in age, blood pressure, and basal metabolic rate.

Another way of examining the question of a relationship between mortality and entry characteristics is to measure the relationships between these characteristics and age at death. Solution of the multiple regression equation with death, age dependent, and fatness independent, found no fatness item to be significant. For all six fatness items together, the correlation with death age was $r = 0.14$ (the square of 0.02 means that only 2% of mortality is "explained" by fatness).

A third way is to consider survival. At the end of follow-up, the youngest men would have been 85 years old, so survival to age 85 years was the target. Death before age 85 years was considered to be lost life years. Solution of the multiple regression equation showed that lost years were not related to fatness but were significantly related to entry age, serum cholesterol, and smoking habit.

FINNS EXAMINED IN 1956 IN THREE AREAS, FOLLOWED FOR 24 YEARS

In the 24-year follow-up of Finns aged 30 to 61 years at entry, among 683 men judged to be healthy at entry, 155 were dead: 71 from coronary artery

TABLE 2. *Numbers of men and deaths, all and coronary, in 40 years in Twin Cities, 24 years in Finns of 1956, in 25 years of five cohorts of the Seven Countries Study, together with means of entry characteristics*

Item	Twin Cities	1956 Finns	East Finland	West Finland	Holland	Crevalcore	Montegiorgio
Number at risk	283	689	694	826	878	993	719
All deaths	219	155	405	420	414	485	327
Coronary	91	71	183	120	171	129	71
Age at entry (years)	49.5	38.2	50.0	50.1	50.0	49.7	49.5
Body mass index	24.9	24.4	24.0	23.3	23.9	25.0	24.4
Systolic BP (mm Hg)	126	136	146	139	144	147	137
Cholesterol (mg/dl)	217	245	268	257	235	202	202

The data for east and west Finland exclude men with CAD at entry.

disease (Table 2). Solution to the multiple logistic equation showed that coronary death was significantly related, *negatively,* to body mass index, positively related to blood pressure and low-density lipoprotein cholesterol, and not significantly related to high-density lipoprotein cholesterol. Mean values of those Finns were as follows: high-density lipoprotein cholesterol, 45.4 mg/dl; low-density lipoprotein cholesterol, 199.3 mg/dl (5–7).

THE SEVEN COUNTRIES STUDY: THE 25-YEAR FOLLOW-UP

For the Seven Countries Study, we consider data for the 25-year follow-up of five cohorts: one in the Netherlands, and two each in Finland and Italy. In the cohorts in Finland, 58 men were also in the 1956 study (3–8). The subjects represented over 97% of the Finns and Italians invited, and 87% of the Dutch. Because coronary artery disease was so prevalent among the Finns, men with evidence of the disease at entry were excluded from the analysis. The exclusions numbered 234 men, 14% of the men in the study, one of seven of all of the men aged 40 to 59 years in the two areas. Among 1,441 of those coronary-free men, 758 men (50%) died in 25 years: 297 from coronary artery disease, 39% of all deaths. Among 878 Dutchmen, 414 died (41% coronary). Among 1,608 Italians, 812 died, 23% from coronary artery disease.

Menotti provided solutions of the Cox proportional hazards equation for coronary death with 12 covariates (Table 3) (9,10). Neither body mass index nor mean skin fold was significant in any cohort. The triceps skinfold was *negatively* significant in one cohort in Italy. Age, blood pressure, and serum cholesterol were positively significant in all cohorts. Physical activity was significantly negatively related to coronary death in all cohorts except in the Netherlands. The

TABLE 3. *Comparison of middle age values and deaths 25 years later, in Seven Countries*

Item	East Finland	West Finland	Zutphen	Crevalcore	Montegiorgio
Age	8.16	7.96	9.90	9.62	8.53
Activity	−1.40	−1.25	−0.37	−0.79	−2.87
Skin folds	−0.85	−1.71	−0.95	−1.66	−2.29
Body mass index	−0.82	1.48	1.04	1.34	2.00
Cholesterol	1.44	−0.39	0.35	1.69	1.22
Cigarettes	5.91	5.28	1.55	3.16	4.07
MBP[a]	6.54	5.68	3.90	5.91	5.53

Cox proportional hazards solutions. *t* values of coefficients.
[a] Mean systolic, diastolic blood pressure.

Finns and the Italians were mostly farmers; the Dutch lived in a small town, most of them in occupations not involving physical work.

Menotti pooled the three national groups for solution of the Cox proportional hazards equation (11). Coronary death was significantly related to age, cholesterol, blood pressure, and smoking and negatively related to activity and arm circumference corrected for skinfold thickness. It is presumed that the corrected arm circumference is a measure of muscle. The pooling may be questioned because of differences among cohorts in habitat, diet, and occupation.

SHORTER PERIODS OF FOLLOW-UP

The relationship of mortality in a relatively short follow-up to characteristics at entry may not be relevant to longevity but it is interesting because most other prospective studies have covered only short periods of follow-up. After 20 years of follow-up, the Twin Cities men were 65 to 75 years old. There had been 71 deaths, 33 coronary. In contrast to the comparison after 40 years, all measures of body fat were significantly lower in the survivors than in the men who died during that period. The difference disappeared after allowance for blood pressure.

Another approach to evaluating the relationships with mortality compares characteristics of men dying relatively early in the follow-up and those dying later. In the Twin Cities study, 114 men died during the first 27 years and 115 men died during the next 13 years. The comparison shows no significant difference in body mass index, skin fold thickness, or relative girth but the men who died relatively early had significantly higher mean blood pressure and serum cholesterol values and were more often cigarette smokers.

In the Seven Countries Study, there were too few coronary deaths in Italy for significant comparison of entry characteristics of coronary dead with survivors in a short follow-up. In Finland and the Netherlands, the 10-year follow-up found age and blood pressure to be significant for coronary and all-causes deaths (4,12). Serum cholesterol was important for coronary but not for all-causes deaths. Cigarette smoking was important in Finland but not in the Netherlands. In the Netherlands, many men smoked cigars instead of cigarettes. In most cohorts, there was no significant linear relationship of mortality to body fat, but there were indications of a possible curvilinear relationship (4,11).

QUESTIONS AND COMMENTS

Some discrepancies between the relationship of mortality to body mass index and to skin fold thickness as measures of fatness in the several cohorts raise questions about the estimation of body fat. A high body mass index could reflect a large muscle mass or a particularly short stature. In regard to skin fold thickness, there are questions as to what sites best indicate body fatness. It has been suggested that central fatness, girth, or the abdominal skin fold thickness, is important. The experience in the Twin Cities Study gives some support to that idea. In the comparisons of men alive with those dead from coronary artery disease after 40 years, the chance probability of a difference is $p = 0.28$ for the triceps skin fold, $p = 0.25$ for the subscapular skin fold, while for the abdominal skinfold it was $p = 0.04$.

Lately, there has been interest in changes of values of risk factors (13). This is important in intervention studies. When there are no large changes, we discuss only characteristics at entry. Temporal changes in the Seven Countries Study are now being analyzed. Changes in populations can be important. We recall the large drop in coronary deaths during the second World War in those countries where the diet changed greatly; meat and fatty foods were very scarce.

Time and the scarcity of data prevent discussion of the direct role of the diet in determining longevity although its importance in regard to serum cholesterol is well established. Also, there has been no discussion of the influence of smoking, which may be different in different populations.

Here, there has been no discussion of nonlinear relationships between mortality and entry characteristics. For the Finns in the Seven Countries Study, there is some indication of a curvilinear relationship between fatness and 25-year mortality from all causes and from coronary artery disease. However, a significant difference between linear and nonlinear relationships of mortality to fatness is hard to prove statistically (14). There is also some question about the form of the relationship of mortality to serum cholesterol.

REFERENCES

1. Keys A. *The cholesterol problem.* Voeding, 1952:539–555.
2. Karvonen MJ, Blomquist G, Kallio V, et al. Men in rural east and west Finland. *Acta Med Scand* 1967;460(suppl):169–190.
3. Keys A. Coronary heart disease in seven countries. *Circulation* 1970;41(suppl 1):1–211.

4. Keys A, Aravanis C, Blackburn H, et al. *Seven Countries Study. A multivariate analysis of death and coronary heart disease.* Cambridge, MA, London: Harvard University Press, 1980:1–381.
5. Keys A, Karvonen MJ, Punsar S, et al. HDL cholesterol and 24-year mortality of men in Finland. *Int J Epidemiol* 1984;13:428–435.
6. Pekkanen J. Coronary heart disease during a 25-year follow-up. Risk factors and their secular trends in the Finnish cohorts of the Seven Countries Study. Health Services Research by the National Board of Health in Finland, 1987.
7. Pekkanen J, Nissinen A, Puska P, et al. Risk factors and 25-year risk of coronary heart disease in a male population with high incidence of the disease. *Br Med J* 1989;299:81–85.
8. Menotti A, Capocaccia R, Farchi G, et al. Stima dell'incidenza di cardiopatia coronarica in una popolazione impiegando la funzione di rischio di un altra. *Rev Lat Cardiol* 1982;3:481–487.
9. Mariotti S, Capocaccia R, Farchi G, et al. Age, period, cohort and geographical effects on coronary heart disease mortality. *J Chron Dis* 1986;39:229–242.
10. Farchi G, Menotti A, Conti S. Coronary risk factors and survival probability from coronary and other causes of death. *Am J Epidemiol* 1987;126:400–408.
11. Menotti A, Keys A, Aravanis C, et al. Seven Countries Study. First 20 years mortality data in 12 cohorts. *Ann Med (Helsinki)* 1989;21:175–189.
12. Nissinen A, Pekkanen J, Porath A, et al. Risk factors for cardiovascular disease among 55 to 74 year-old Finnish men. A 10-year follow-up. *Ann Med (Helsinki)* 1989;21:239–240.
13. Blackburn H. Population strategies of cardiovascular disease prevention. Scientific base, rationale and public health implications. *Ann Med (Helsinki)* 1989;21:157–162.
14. Keys A. Longevity of man. Relative weight and fatness in middle age. *Ann Med (Helsinki)* 1989;21:163–168.

Atherosclerosis Reviews, Volume 21,
edited by A. Leaf and P. C. Weber.
Raven Press, Ltd., New York © 1990.

Serum Lipids and Risk of Coronary Artery Disease

William P. Castelli, Peter W. F. Wilson,
Daniel Levy, and Keaven Anderson

Framingham Heart Study, Framingham, Massachusetts 01701

In the U.S., slightly less than one-half the men and women die from a degenerative vascular disease related to atherosclerosis. This process causes heart attacks and strokes and other vascular problems. Long before they die from this disease, one-third of the men and women will experience a clinical episode of this disease. Evidence will be examined from the prospective study of a free living population in Framingham, Massachusetts relating the measurement of various measures of blood fats, from simple measures such as the total cholesterol to examination of the role of the various lipoproteins such as low-density lipoproteins (LDL), very low-density lipoproteins (VLDL or triglycerides), and high-density lipoproteins (HDL) in the genesis of coronary artery disease (CAD), which represents about two-thirds of the clinical manifestations of atherosclerosis. A large proportion of the people destined to get coronary artery disease can be identified many years prior to their illness so that a short comment will be made addressing the evidence that lowering blood cholesterol will lower the subsequent rate of this disease.

METHODS

In 1948, the Framingham Heart Study began the recruitment of 5,209 men and women for the study. Of these, 5,127 were found to be free of CAD and other vascular diseases at entry. Seven-eighths of these people were selected randomly from the 10,000 men and women living in Framingham at the time. Many things were measured in these people throughout the more than 40 years of this study; subjects were examined every 2 years to ascertain whether they had developed CAD or other vascular or other diseases in the interim. Coronary artery disease was diagnosed as one of the following: angina pectoris, coronary insufficiency, myocardial infarction, and coronary artery disease death, sudden or nonsudden by protocols previously described (1). Blood cholesterols were measured by the method of Abell and Kendall (2) and lipoproteins were originally measured in the analytical ultracentrifuge by Gofman (3), and more recently by protocols developed for the Lipids Research Clinic Program (4).

RESULTS

The total serum cholesterol shows a curvilinear relationship with CAD in men and women at ages 35–84 years. In each 10-year age span, the relative impact is greater in younger men than in older men, but the absolute rate of disease is worse in older men. If one pools the data over and under age 50 years, this relationship is statistically significant on multivariate analysis taking into account age, sex, blood pressure, cigarette smoking, diabetes, and left ventricular hypertrophy on ECG at $p = 0.001$ in women at all ages and in the younger

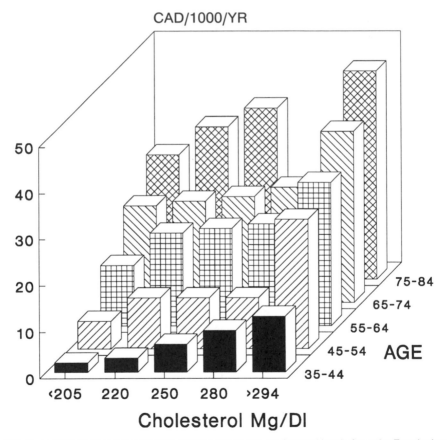

FIG. 1. Incidence of coronary artery disease in men vs. cholesterol levels from the Framingham Heart Study (30-year data). From ref. 6.

men. It is significant at $p = 0.04$ in the older men when the follow-up is carried out to 12 years instead of 2 years, as shown in Figs. 1 and 2 (5,6). Notice that the relationship of cholesterol to CAD in women in Fig. 2 does differ from that for men in that the absolute rates of CAD appear to be very low prior to age 50 years, the age of menopause. It is after 50 years of age that women really start to catch up to men. Eventually, just as many women will develop CAD as men; in older women, both the relative and absolute impact of cholesterol is greater than in younger women.

The total cholesterol is carried in our blood in five major lipoproteins: chylomicrons, very-low-density lipoproteins, intermediate-density lipoproteins, low-density lipoproteins, and high-density lipoproteins. Three of these (VLDL, LDL, and HDL) have been studied extensively in Framingham. Figure 3 shows that in men and women, the LDL as measured at entry in the analytical ultra-

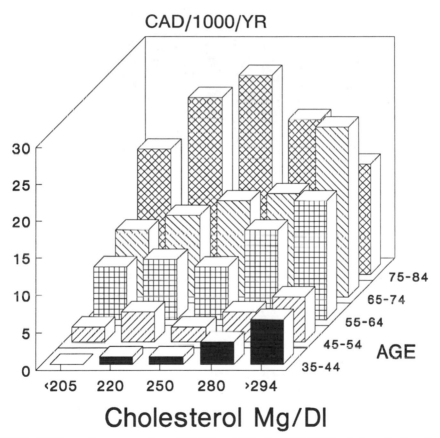

FIG. 2. Incidence of coronary artery disease in women vs. cholesterol levels from the Framingham Heart Study (30-year data). From ref. 6.

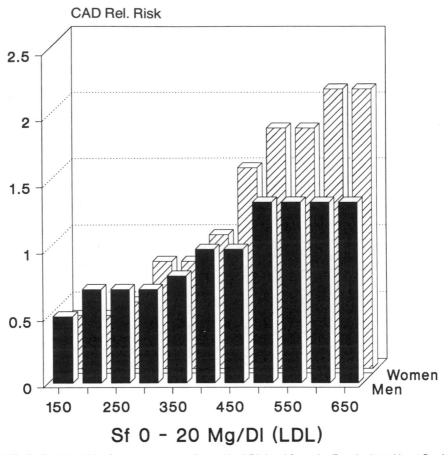

FIG. 3. Relative risk of coronary artery disease by LDL level from the Framingham Heart Study (30-year follow-up). From ref. 6.

centrifuge is related to CAD. VLDL, where most of the triglycerides are carried, is also related to CAD in men and women in an almost linear fashion (Fig. 4). However, on multivariate analysis where LDL has been an independent risk factor, it has only been so for triglycerides in women (7). This has caused some to discard triglycerides in men as an important factor (8). However, there are problems with the mathematical models used in these analyses. For one, they assumed that VLDLs were homogeneous and that as they rose it was only a quantitative change and could be used as a continuous variable. Recent data from many sources such as Steiner (9) and Schonfeld (10) suggest that when triglycerides rise, there is a production of smaller, denser VLDLs that are cleared less readily from blood and lead to overproduction of LDLs that are also smaller and denser and may be more atherogenic (11). Rather than adjust triglycerides

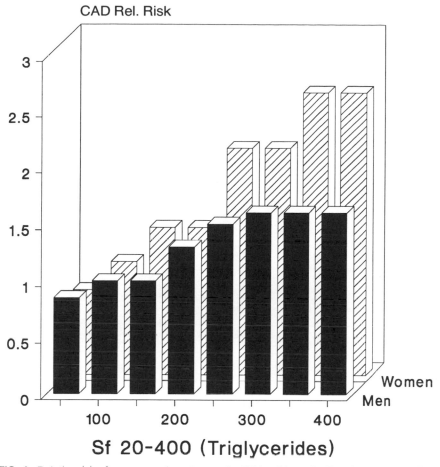

FIG. 4. Relative risk of coronary artery disease by TG level from the Framingham Heart Study (30-year follow-up). From ref. 6.

by HDL in statistical models, it would appear that there is more to be learned by stratifying triglycerides by HDL, as seen in Figs. 5 and 6. In both instances, there is a subgroup of subjects with high triglycerides (over 150 mg/dl) and low HDL (under 40 mg/dl) who have higher rates of CAD than any of the other subgroups. These "high triglyceride" people also tend to have higher blood sugars and uric acids (Figs. 7 and 8). Recently, Reaven (12) has described increased insulin resistance and hypertension in these people, a combination he unfortunately called syndrome "X." Since we already have a syndrome "X" in cardiology, perhaps we should call it "Reaven's syndrome." Williams and his colleagues in Salt Lake City have found this syndrome to run in families and they call it "familial dyslipidemic hypertension" (13). Triglycerides have also been

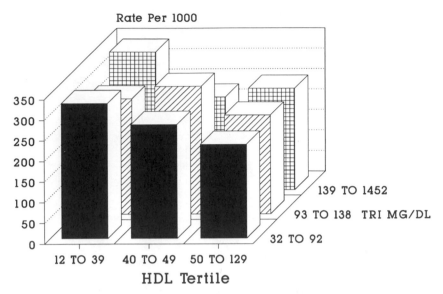

FIG. 5. Incidence of CAD by triglyceride and HDL levels, age-adjusted 14-year rates in men. Age range at baseline was 50 to 84 years. From ref. 6.

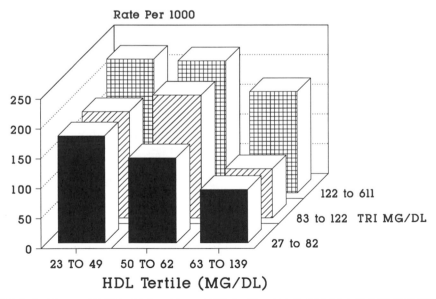

FIG. 6. Incidence of CAD by triglyceride and HDL levels, age-adjusted 14-year rates in women. Age range at baseline was 50 to 84 years. From ref. 6.

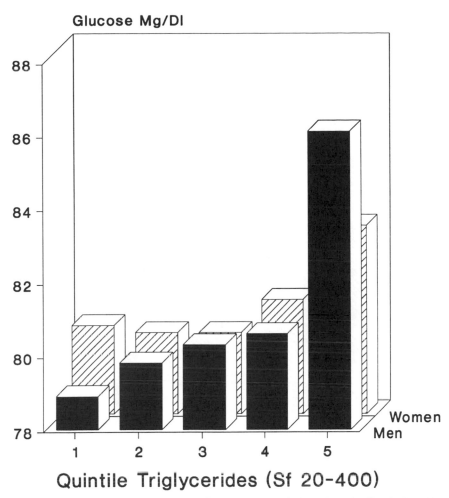

FIG. 7. Blood sugar vs. triglyceride levels, linear model correlations, from the Framingham Heart Study. From ref. 6.

described as independent risk factors in Sweden (14) and the risk from a subgroup of people with high triglycerides has been described from the Lipid Research Clinics Program (15). Autopsy studies have also shown an independent effect of triglycerides on lesion mass (16,17).

HDL cholesterol is inversely related to CAD in men and in women (Fig. 9). This relationship is the strongest in statistical terms for any other lipid particle studied so far. It is both independently (on multivariate analysis) and powerfully (on likelihood ratio analysis) related to risk.

The bulk of the heart attacks in Framingham occur in men and women who have total cholesterols between 200 and 240 mg/dl (5.2 and 6.2 mmol, respec-

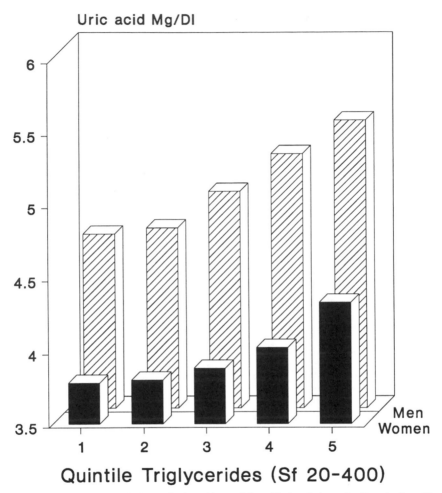

Uric acid Mg/Dl

Quintile Triglycerides (Sf 20-400)

FIG. 8. Linear model correlations of uric acid vs. triglyceride levels from the Framingham Heart Study. From ref. 6.

tively). Twenty percent of CAD develops in subjects with a total cholesterol under 200 mg/dl. Figure 10 shows that the best way to identify the people under 200 mg/dl who are running an inordinate risk is to measure their HDL. If their HDLs are less than 40 mg/dl, then they are running the same risk as individuals with total cholesterols in the 230 to 300+ mg/dl range. HDL is also the best predictor in people who have a total cholesterol between 200 and 240 mg/dl of who is headed for a heart attack. It is a two to three times more powerful predictor than is the LDL cholesterol in this range. In persons with cholesterol levels over 250 mg/dl, LDL cholesterol becomes a much better predictor but occasionally a person with a very high HDL will be found with a ratio of total choles-

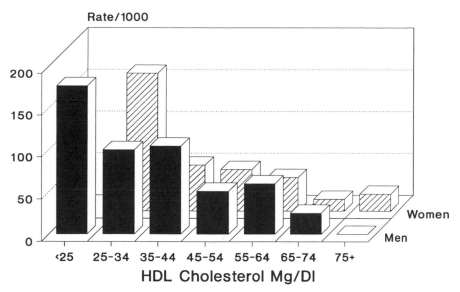

FIG. 9. Incidence of coronary artery disease vs. HDL cholesterol levels. From ref. 7.

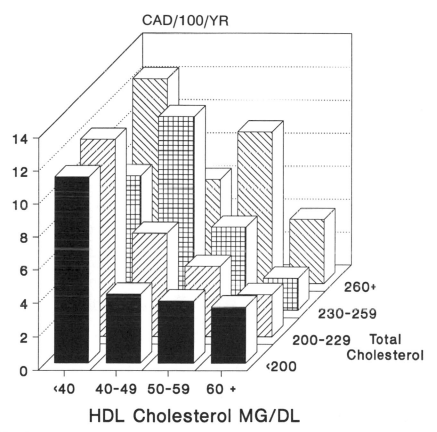

FIG. 10. Incidence of coronary artery disease by total and HDL cholesterol levels in subjects aged 50 to 79 years. From ref. 5.

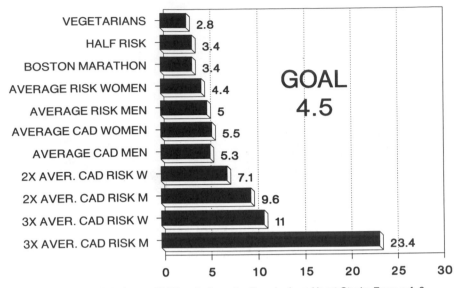

FIG. 11. Total cholesterol/HDL ratio from the Framingham Heart Study. From ref. 6.

terol to HDL cholesterol of under 3.5, which is a very safe profile. In older subjects over age 60 years, HDL provides the most power to predict who will develop CAD and therefore needs therapy.

Figure 11 shows the total cholesterol/HDL cholesterol ratio. Risk is very high once one exceeds a ratio of 4.5. About one-half of Americans have such a ratio and almost all of these people get this disease, so we are recommending that a ratio of 4.5 be used as a goal of therapy. An ideal ratio is probably under 3.5. If the total cholesterol falls to 150 mg/dl or below, it is not necessary to know the HDL; once your cholesterol exceeds 150 mg/dl, it is a good practice to find out what the patient's LDL, triglyceride, and HDL levels are to find people with serious lipid problems.

DISCUSSION

The total cholesterol level gives us the opportunity to see that lipids continue to predict risk of CAD to a very old age but the breakdown of the total cholesterol into LDL, triglyceride, and HDL cholesterols allows a more precise definition of which individuals run an inordinate risk. The National Cholesterol Education Program has recently set goals of therapy for cholesterol treatment (diet and drug): LDL cholesterols under 160 mg/dl or under 130 mg/dl if the person already has vascular disease or two of the following risk factors: male, family history, under 55 years of age, HDL under 35 mg/dl, smoking, hypertension, obesity, or diabetes. We would add that the ratio must be under 4.5.

One can add to the identification of risk the knowledge in practically every diet (Fig. 12) and drug (Fig. 13) trial done that the lower the cholesterol level, the lower the subsequent rate of CAD. One must tie the CAD response to the fall in cholesterol to maintain the logic of such a sequence.

Cholesterol is not the only risk factor; however, it is a factor that must be understood in its entirety if the people with dangerous levels are to be found and thereby helped. Far too many people think it is only necessary to treat people with cholesterol levels of 300 mg/dl or more, but the average man in Framingham who develops CAD has a cholesterol level of 225 mg/dl. If we are to do something about the current epidemic of atherosclerotic disease, we must

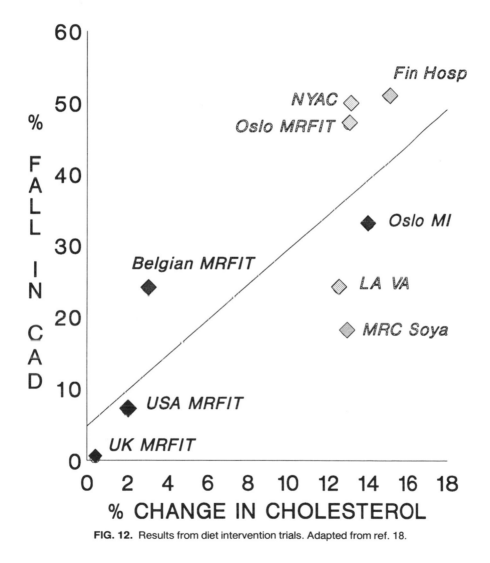

FIG. 12. Results from diet intervention trials. Adapted from ref. 18.

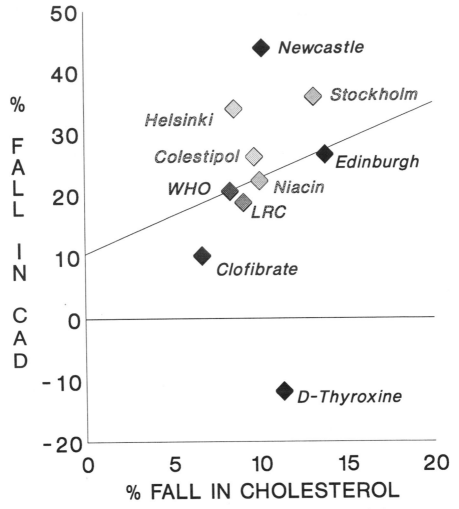

FIG. 13. Results from drug intervention trials. Adapted from ref. 18.

find the high-risk people with cholesterol levels between 200 and 240 mg/dl. The best way to do this is to measure HDL, and then LDL and triglycerides. In addition, it is important to know the patient's blood pressure, smoking status, blood sugar, weight, exercise pattern, etc. Over 90% of people with cholesterols at 300 mg/dl or higher will go on in the next 30 years to develop CAD; to do a good job of finding a high-risk group between 200 and 240 mg/dl, one needs to add all of the other major risk factors into the equation. However, unlike the 300 mg/dl cholesterol group, very few of the 200–240 mg/dl group will need anything other than a good hygienic program (diet and exercise) to control their risks and thereby their destiny.

Finally, there is a groundswell of evidence implicating a syndrome involving high triglycerides (over 150 mg/dl), low HDL cholesterol (under 40 mg/dl), high blood sugar, increased insulin resistance, increased girth, and increased uric acid in the genesis of coronary artery disease. These people frequently have unimpressive total and LDL cholesterols, but they have accelerated rates of atherogenesis.

REFERENCES

1. Abbott RD, McGee D. The probability of developing certain cardiovascular diseases in eight years: specified values of some characteristics. National Heart, Lung, and Blood Institute, U.S. Dept. of Health and Human Services, NIH Publication No. 87-2284.
2. Abell LL, Levy BB, Brodie BB, Kendall FB. A simplified method for the estimation of total cholesterol in serum and demonstration of its specificity. *J Biol Chem* 1952;195:357–366.
3. Gofman JW, Young W, Tandy R. Ischemic heart disease, atherosclerosis, and longevity. *Circulation* 1966;34:79.
4. Lipid Research Clinics Program. *Manual of laboratory operations. Vol. 1. Lipid and lipoprotein analysis,* DHEW Publication No. (NIH) 75-628. Bethesda, MD: National Institutes of Health, 1976.
5. Castelli WP, Garrison RJ, Wilson PWF, Abbott RD, Kalousdian S, Kannel WB. Incidence of coronary heart disease and lipoprotein cholesterol levels. The Framingham Study. *JAMA* 1986;256:2835–2838.
6. Castelli WP. Cholesterol and lipids in the risk of coronary artery disease—The Framingham Heart Study. *Can J Cardiol* 1988;4(suppl A):5A–10A.
7. Gordon T, Castelli WP, Hjortland MC, Kannel WB, Dawber TR. High density lipoprotein as a protective factor against coronary heart disease. The Framingham Study. *Am J Med* 1977;62: 707–714.
8. Hulley SB, Rosenham RH, Bawol RD, Brond RJ. Epidemiology as a guide to clinical decisions: the association between triglyceride and coronary heart disease. *N Engl J Med* 1980;302:1383–1389.
9. Poapst M, Reardon M, Steiner G. Relative contribution of triglyceride-rich lipoprotein particle size and number to plasma triglyceride concentration. *Arteriosclerosis* 1985;5:381–390.
10. Schonfeld G. Disorders of lipid transport—update 1983. *Prog Cardiovasc Dis* 1983;26:89–108.
11. Sniderman AD, Wolfson C, Teng B, Franklin FA, Bachorik PS, Kwiterovitch PO Jr. Association of hyperapobetalipoproteinemia with endogenous hypertriglyceridemia and atherosclerosis. *Ann Intern Med* 1982;63:833–839.
12. Reaven GM. The role of insulin resistance in human disease. *Diabetes* 1988;37:1595–1607.
13. Williams RR, Hunt SC, Hopkins PN, et al. Familial dyslipidemic hypertension: evidence from 58 Utah families for a syndrome present in approximately 12% of patients with essential hypertension. *JAMA* 1988;259:3579–3586.
14. Bottiger LE, Carlson LA. Risk factors for ischaemic vascular death for men in the Stockholm prospective study. *Atherosclerosis* 1980;36:389.
15. Criqui M, Heiss G, Cohn R, Cowan LD, Suchindran CM, Bangdiwala S. Triglycerides and coronary heart disease mortality. The Lipid Research Clinics Follow-Up Study. *CVD Epidemiol Newslett* 1987;41:13.
16. Reardon MF, Nestel PJ, Craig IH, Harper RW. Lipoprotein predictors of the severity of coronary artery disease in men and women. *Circulation* 1985;71:881–888.
17. Cabin HS, Roberts WC. Relation of serum total cholesterol and triglycerides to the amount and extent of coronary arterial narrowing by atherosclerotic plaque in coronary heart disease. Quantitative analysis of 2037 five mm segments of 160 major epicardial coronary arteries in 40 necropsy patients. *Am J Med* 1982;73:227.
18. The Lipid Research Clinic Program. The Lipid Research Clinics Coronary Primary Prevention Trial results: II. The relationship of reduction in incidence of coronary heart disease to cholesterol lowering. *JAMA* 1984;251:365–374.

Atherosclerosis Reviews, Volume 21,
edited by A. Leaf and P. C. Weber.
Raven Press, Ltd., New York © 1990.

Diet and Ischemic Heart Disease in Japan

Yuichiro Goto and Emilio H. Moriguchi

Department of Medicine, Tokai University School of Medicine,
Bohseidai, Isehara-shi, Kanagawa-ken 259-11, Japan

Traditionally the incidence of myocardial infarction has been substantially lower in Japan than it is in the industrialized west (Fig. 1). Generally it has been thought that this is related, in part, to the lower serum cholesterol levels among the Japanese people, and this has been attributed, in turn, to diet (Fig. 2). Over the past few decades, however, the incidence of ischemic heart disease (IHD) in Japan has increased. It is postulated that this change parallels changes in diet and lipid levels (Fig. 3) (1).

TRENDS IN THE DIET, SERUM LIPID LEVELS, AND IHD IN JAPAN

Japanese lifestyle has become westernized since World War II and, as a result, so have the Japanese dietary habits (Fig. 4). In 1949, average Japanese diets contained 81% of total energy of the diet (en%) as carbohydrate with 7-en% as fat. In 1960, carbohydrates accounted for 76.1-en% and fat for almost 11-en%. In 1987, only 60-en% were provenient from carbohydrates and almost 25-en% from fat. The speed with which Japanese diets have changed is reflected in the 1988 report that the average diet of 10- to 11-year-old Japanese girls consisted of 50-en% carbohydrate with 34-en% fat (2), values that approach those of the current typical American diet. Careful and more detailed analysis of the nutritional data from the Ministry of Health and Welfare of Japan (3) shows the following:

In the last 35 years, the proportion of the nutrients as energy in the Japanese diet has suffered gradual but steady changes: whereas energy from carbohydrates decreased from almost 80-en% in 1955 to <60-en% in 1987, fat increased its participation in diet from 8.7-en% in 1955 to almost 25-en% in 1987 with no significant changes in the total calorie intake (Fig. 5).

The daily intake of protein in Japan increased from <70 g per capita in 1955 to almost 82 g in 1975 and now fluctuates around 80 g. In 1955, animal protein was responsible for less than one-third of the total protein intake, but

21

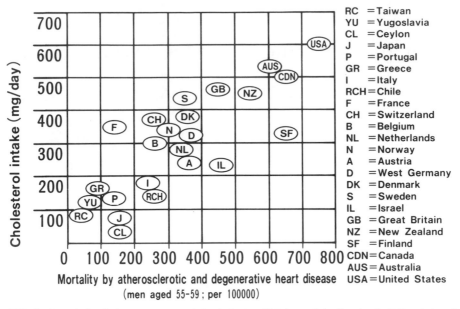

FIG. 1. Correlation between average daily cholesterol intake and deaths due to ischemic heart disease. From ref. 9.

its presence has increased steadily and now >50% of the protein of the Japanese diet is of animal origin (Fig. 6).

Inseparable from those dietary changes are the modifications in the fat intake: The daily intake of fat was 28.3 g per capita in 1955, and after increasing yearly it reached 56.6 g in 1987, exactly twice its 1955 value. Similar to protein intake, animal fats were responsible for less than one-third of the total fat intake in 1955, but now almost 50% of the fat is of animal origin (Fig. 7).

Changes in nutrient intake in Japan in the last 40 years can be reiterated as follows (Fig. 8):

The total energy intake increased at the end of the 1940s until it reached a plateau during the early 1950s; it now shows a decrease starting at the beginning of the 1970s.

Carbohydrates in the diet as an energy source have decreased steadily by about 20% in the last 30 years.

Total protein intake had increased gradually by about 30% until the early 1970s when it reached a peak and afterward decreased slightly.

The intake of animal protein increased more than 3.5-fold until it peaked during the early 1970s; since then those high intake values have been maintained.

Total fat intake had increased also more than 3.5-fold until the end of the 1970s and has maintained those high levels. The intake of animal fat increased more than fivefold until the early 1970s and has maintained those high levels also.

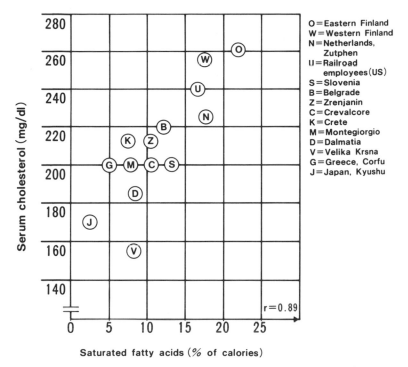

FIG. 2. Correlation between total cholesterol and the proportion of saturated fatty acids in the diet. From ref. 9.

What happened to the dietary habits of the Japanese people that resulted in such a modification of nutrient intake? The data from the Ministry of Health and Welfare of Japan show that in the last 30 years, while the intake of components of the Japanese traditional diet (e.g., rice, beans, and some vegetables) has decreased, the intake of components of the Western diet (such as meats, eggs, milk, and dairy products) has increased tremendously. Although fish (rich in polyunsaturated fatty acids of the *n*-3 group) consists of animal protein, its consumption has not increased significantly; rather the presence of fish as a proportion of the whole and daily Japanese diet has decreased (Fig. 9).

As can be seen, the dietary habits in Japan are becoming rapidly similar to those in the USA: increasing in protein intake, decreasing in carbohydrates, increasing in fat intake, and decreasing in polyunsaturated/saturated fatty acids and *n*-3/*n*-6 ratios (Fig. 10).

As is observed with Japanese who emigrate to Hawaii and California and whose changed dietary patterns result in negative health consequences [i.e., an increased intake of total fat, saturated fat, and cholesterol resulting in an increase in the incidence of ischemic heart disease (Table 1)], the increasing west-

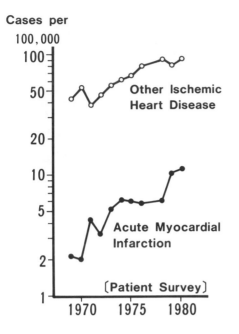

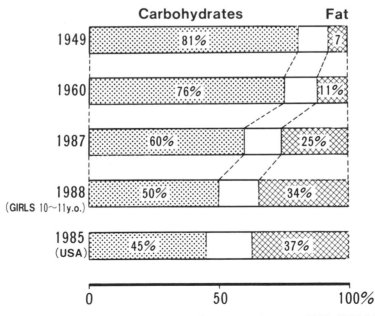

FIG. 3. Incidence of ischemic heart diseases in Japan. From ref. 3.

FIG. 4. Trends of intake of carbohydrates and fat in Japan between 1949–1988 (% of total energy). From ref. 3.

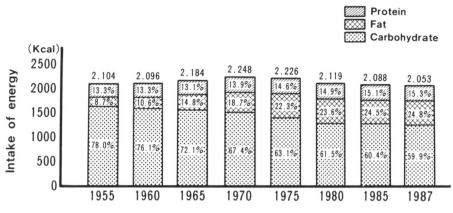

FIG. 5. Trends of intake of energy per capita per day in Japan. From ref. 3.

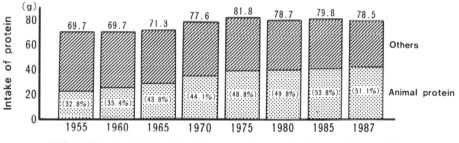
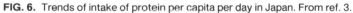

FIG. 6. Trends of intake of protein per capita per day in Japan. From ref. 3.

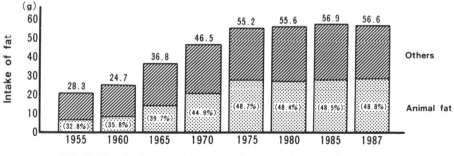
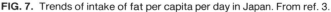

FIG. 7. Trends of intake of fat per capita per day in Japan. From ref. 3.

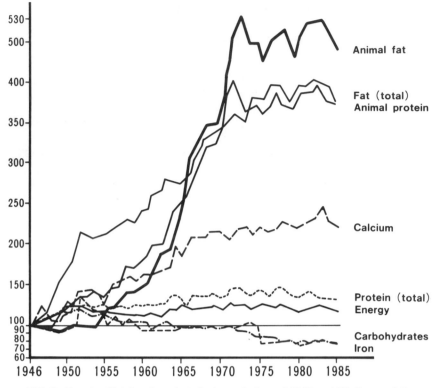

FIG. 8. Trends of intake of nutrients in Japan (values of 1946 as 100). From ref. 3.

ernization of the Japanese diet and lifestyle has changed patterns of macronutrient consumption, leading to a "shift" in the incidence of diseases to the "Western side" (Fig. 11).

It is important to stress that those changes in Japanese dietary habits have brought not only negative results, but also some positive ones: for example, the dramatic reduction in Japanese death due to cerebrovascular diseases (Fig. 12) illustrates an important successful nationwide effort to decrease salt intake (Fig. 13). Salt-preserved foods, abundant in the traditional Japanese diet, might have played an etiologic role also in the high incidence of stomach cancer, which has been linked epidemiologically to cerebral hemorrhage or stroke. Thus, benefits clearly occurred in voluntarily changing from the previous to the present Japanese diet and lifestyle because these diseases decreased.

However, the increasing incidence of heart diseases, mainly ischemic heart disease (IHD), is worrisome (Fig. 14). The mortality rate of IHD increased from 10 per 100,000 in 1949 to >40 in the early 1980s, accounting for 40% of the total deaths due to heart disease (4). We have postulated that this change parallels changes in diet and serum lipid levels (1).

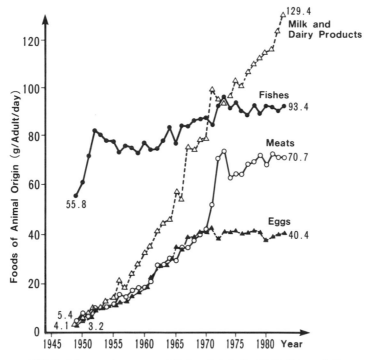

FIG. 9. Changes in average daily food intake in Japan. From ref. 3.

Since the 1960s, we have made sequential observations of serum lipids of a large number of Japanese people (5–7). In 1961, the average serum cholesterol level studied in 6,977 normal subjects was 176 mg/dl. The second survey, made in 1970 on 3,555 subjects, revealed that the averages were 185 mg/dl for men and 187 mg/dl for women. The third survey, conducted from 1980 to 1981 on 10,977 subjects, demonstrated that the mean cholesterol level increased to 190 mg/dl for men and 192 mg/dl for women, showing an increase of approximately 15 mg/dl from 1961 to 1981 (Fig. 15). The fourth survey is being conducted currently, and we expect further increases in the cholesterol level of Japanese people.

Comparing the serum cholesterol levels of Japanese subjects in the 1980s with Americans during the middle 1970s, it is worth noting that Japanese cholesterol levels are much higher in the 1980s than were American levels in the 1970s for both males and females < 30 years of age (Fig. 16).

It is well known that serum cholesterol levels have a direct correlation with the incidence of IHD. The mortality rate from myocardial infarction is still lower in Japanese than it is in Americans; however, it is possible that these rates can increase within 10 to 20 years if the young Japanese do not change their dietary habits now.

	Japan 1960 %	Japan 1985 %	U.S.A 1985 %
Proteins	13	14	16
Carbohydrates	75	61	45
Fats	11	25	37
Saturated	3	8	14
Monounsaturated	4	9	15
Polyunsaturated	4	8	8
n-3/n-6	0.34	0.26	0.12

FIG. 10. Changes in dietary patterns in Japan compared to USA. From ref. 10.

Results of a nation-wide cooperative study (Japanese) published last year (8) of atherosclerosis in young, first-generation Japanese ranging in age from 1 month to 39 years confirm our fears: Japanese infants, children, and young adults already present atherosclerotic lesions early in life at a rate similar to that of the U.S.A. This study shows the startling data that even in infants under 1 year of age fatty streaks are seen in 28.8% of aortas, accounting for approximately 3% of the intimal surface in the mean value (Fig. 17). In the coronary arteries, lesions are found at an early age also and, by the age of 10, fatty streaks are present in 3.1% of coronary arteries (Fig. 18). In both cases, the presence of fatty streaks increased rapidly in the second decade of life, compared to that prior to the age of 10. In the second decade of life, progression of these streaks slowed and reached a plateau thereafter. Now, however, instead of fatty streaks, fibrous plaques gradually increased within the arteries after the third decade. Correlation of antemortem clinical data with the localization and severity of atherosclerotic lesions showed that for both the aorta and coronary arteries,

TABLE 1. *Changes in dietary habits of Japanese men following emigration to Hawaii or California and the influence on serum cholesterol and incidence of ischemic heart disease (IHD)*

	Japan	Hawaii	California
Total calories	2,164 ± 619	2,275 ± 736	2,262 ± 695
Animal protein (g)	39.8 ± 22.8	70.5 ± 32.7	66.0 ± 24.4
Total fat (g)	36.6 ± 20.4	85.1 ± 38.9	94.8 ± 36.4
Saturated fat (g)	16.0 ± 13.3	59.1 ± 32.7	66.3 ± 30.5
Cholesterol (mg)	464.1 ± 324.4	545.1 ± 316.4	533.2 ± 297.8
Serum cholesterol (mg/dl)	181.1 ± 38.5	218.3 ± 38.2	228.2 ± 42.2
Number per 1,000 >260 mg/dl	31.6	124.0	162.5
Myocardial infarction and death due to IHD. Incidence compared to Japanese men in Japan	—	Twofold	Threefold

From ref. 9.

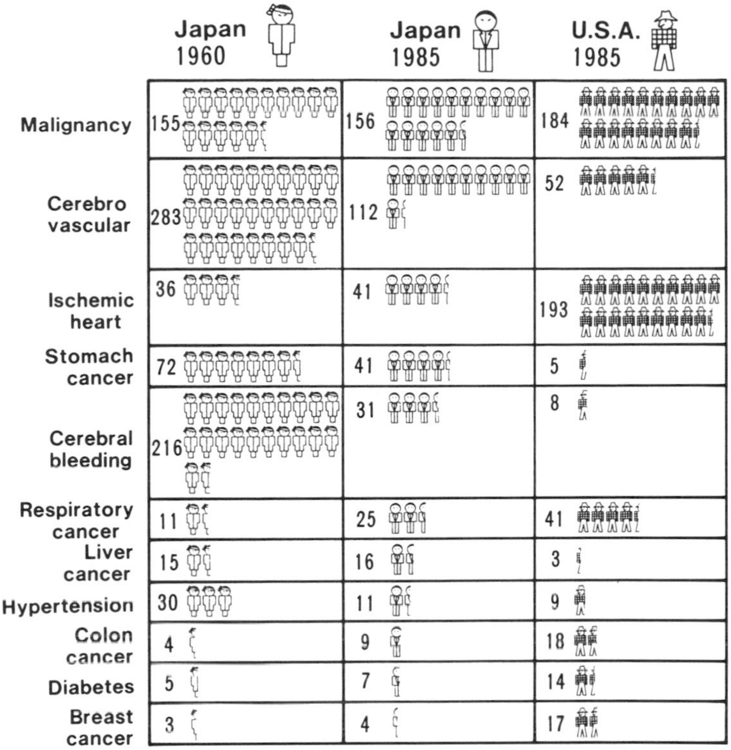

	Japan 1960	Japan 1985	U.S.A. 1985
Malignancy	155	156	184
Cerebro vascular	283	112	52
Ischemic heart	36	41	193
Stomach cancer	72	41	5
Cerebral bleeding	216	31	8
Respiratory cancer	11	25	41
Liver cancer	15	16	3
Hypertension	30	11	9
Colon cancer	4	9	18
Diabetes	5	7	14
Breast cancer	3	4	17

FIG. 11. Death rates from specific diseases (age- and sex-adjusted per 100,000 of 1985 Japanese population). From ref. 10.

serum cholesterol was a strong factor for progression of fatty streaks, whereas mean blood pressure was a strong factor for the progression of fibrous plaques: both risk factors are diet-dependent.

FINAL COMMENTS

To a certain extent, traditional dietary patterns in Japan are not evident. Because Japanese diets have changed dramatically in the last 40 years, it is inappropriate to assume that the pattern of macronutrients that characterized traditional Japanese diets has been maintained in current Japanese diets. The westernization of the Japanese diet and lifestyle has changed patterns of macronutrient consumption, yielding negative health consequences. Fortunately, there was a reduction in the incidence of cerebrovascular diseases, although

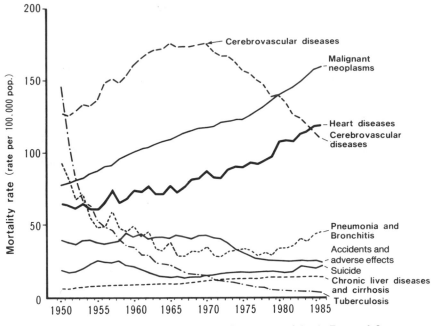

FIG. 12. Trends of death rates by leading causes of death. From ref. 3.

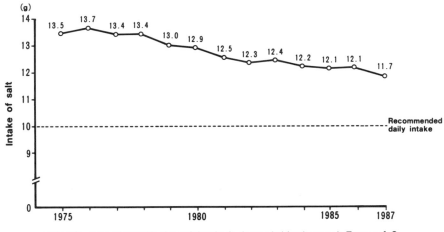

FIG. 13. Annual trend in the salt intake in Japan (g/day/person). From ref. 3.

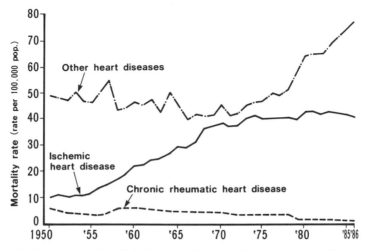

FIG. 14. Annual trend of mortality from heart diseases by types in Japan. From ref. 3.

the incidence of cardiovascular diseases, mainly of ischemic heart disease, has increased. Unfortunately, the incidence of ischemic heart disease in Japan may continue to increase in the near future, and it might be due to increasing serum cholesterol levels from the changes in the dietary habits. Because of this, we are instituting programs for dietary education, particularly for young Japanese people, to prevent further increases in cholesterol levels and in the incidence of ischemic heart disease.

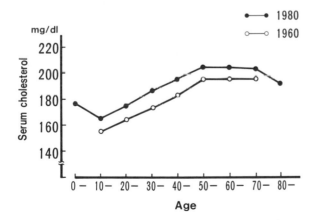

FIG. 15. Changes in serum cholesterol levels in Japan. From ref. 1.

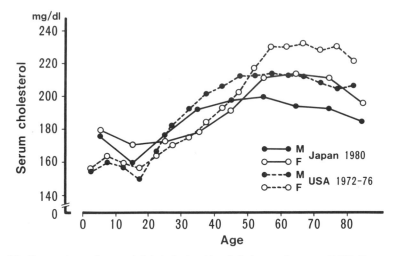

FIG. 16. Comparison of serum total cholesterol levels between Japan and USA. From ref. 6.

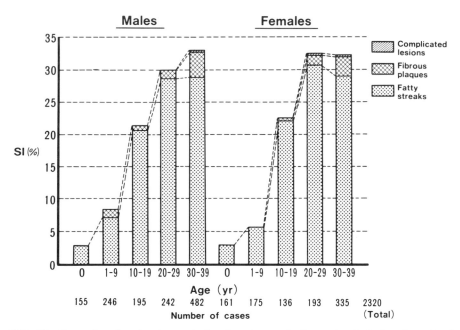

FIG. 17. Mean of surface involvement of various types of atherosclerotic lesions in aortas in infants, children, and young adults in Japan. From ref. 8.

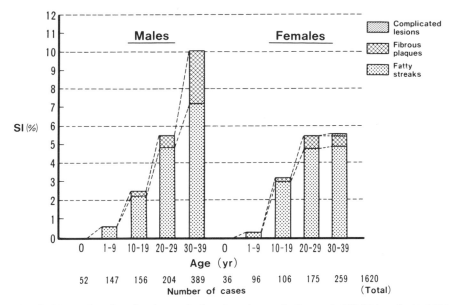

FIG. 18. Mean of surface involvement of various types of atherosclerotic lesions in coronary arteries in infants, children, and young adults in Japan. From ref. 8.

REFERENCES

1. Goto Y. Cholesterol level of Japanese in past twenty years and primary prevention study by dextran sulfate (MDS). In: Fidge NH, Nestel PJ, eds. *Atherosclerosis VII.* Amsterdam: Elsevier. 1986:9–14.
2. Nakajima H, Sueyoshi Y, Kikuchi F, et al. The relationship between the nutritional intake and serum lipids of children in Numazu city [in Japanese]. *Shouni Hoken Kenkyu* 1988;47:657–668.
3. Health Statistics Association. Patients and medical institutions in Japan—graphic view of health statistics [in Japanese]. Tokyo: Ministry of Health and Welfare of Japan, 1989.
4. Goto Y, Homma Y. Recent trends of coronary heart disease in Japan in relation to dietary alterations. In: Yamori Y, ed. *Nutritional prevention of cardiovascular disease.* San Diego: Academic Press. 1984:73–85.
5. Goto Y. Epidemiology and prevention of atherosclerotic diseases [in Japanese]. *Igaku to Yakugaku* 1981;6:567–74.
6. Sekimoto H, Goto Y, Goto Y, et al. Changes of serum total cholesterol and triglyceride levels in normal subjects in Japan in the past twenty years. *Jpn Circ J* 1983;47:1351–1358.
7. Goto Y. Serum cholesterol and nutrition in Japan. *Jpn J Med* 1986;25:113.
8. Tanaka K, et al. A nation-wide study of atherosclerosis in infants, children and young adults in Japan. *Atherosclerosis* 1988;72:143–156.
9. Assmann G. *Lipid metabolism and atherosclerosis.* Stuttgart: Schattauer, 1982:246 pp.
10. Lands WEM, Hamazaki T, Yamazaki K, et al. A story of changing dietary patterns. *Am J Clin Nutr* 1990 (in press).

Atherosclerosis Reviews, Volume 21,
edited by A. Leaf and P. C. Weber.
Raven Press, Ltd., New York © 1990.

Physical Activity, Physical Fitness, and Coronary Heart Disease

Ralph S. Paffenbarger, Jr.

*Department of Health Research and Policy, Stanford University
School of Medicine, Stanford, California 94305-5092*

The past decade has seen general acceptance of epidemiological evidence that physical activity promotes physical fitness and counters tendencies toward development of coronary heart disease (CHD). This study presents a brief overview of salient observations to support this concept.

PHYSICAL ACTIVITY

Table 1 shows the findings of three epidemiological studies of the influences of leisure-time physical activity on the relative risks of CHD among populations in England and the United States. The 7,820 British men cited in the top panel of the table were middle-aged, middle-class, executive-grade civil servants who largely were confined to desk jobs and variously inclined to devote some of their leisure hours to physically vigorous recreational sports and hobbies (1–3). After being queried in 1976 about how many episodes of vigorous exercise they had indulged in during the previous month, such as sportsplay requiring expenditure of at least 7.5 kcal/min, they were followed until 1985 for incidence of CHD. Only 4% reported eight or more sessions of vigorous exercise per month by postal questionnaire, but their risk of CHD during the follow-up interval was barely one-third that of men who reported no such exercise. A consistent gradient of benefit was seen between these extremes.

The second panel of Table 1 shows a similar but less striking trend of risk associated with tri-levels of a daily physical activity index derived from interviewing 12,138 middle-aged U.S. Multiple Risk Factor Intervention Trial (MRFIT) men who were considered to be at relatively high risk of developing CHD because of their serum lipoprotein profiles and blood pressure levels, cigarette-smoking habits, and weight-for-height status (4). Although their exercise patterns were at best moderate by most standards, the most active third were twice as energetic as the middle third, who in turn were twice as active as the lowest third, in terms of kilocalories expended per day. During the follow-up interval, 1976 to 1985, their CHD rates per 100 men ranged about the same as was noted

TABLE 1. *Relative risks of coronary heart disease (CHD) by levels of physical activity in selected populations*

British civil servants[a]	Sessions of vigorous sports in past 4 weeks	% of men	CHD rate per 100 men[d]	Relative risk of CHD
9-yr follow-up,	0	83	6.3	1.00
1976–1985	1–3	8	5.1	0.81
	4–7	5	3.6	0.57
	8+	4	2.0	0.32
Multiple risk factor interventional trial[b]	Tertiles of physical activity in kcal/day		CHD rate per 100 men[e]	Relative risk of CHD
8-yr follow-up,	Low		7.2	1.00
1973–1981	Moderate		6.4	0.88
	High		5.8	0.81
Harvard alumni[c]	Physical activity index in kcal/week	% of man–yrs	CHD rate per 1,000 man–yr[f]	Relative risk of CHD
10-yr follow-up,	<2,000	62	5.8	1.00
1962–1972	2,000+	38	3.5	0.61

[a] 7,820 men, ages 45 to 59 years at entry.
[b] 12,138 men, 35–57 at entry.
[c] 16,936 men, ages 35 to 74 years at entry.
[d] Adjusted for age-differences; $p = 0.03$.
[e] Adjusted for age-differences; $p < 0.01$.
[f] Adjusted for differences in age, cigarette habit, and blood-pressure status; $p < 0.01$.

above for the least active British civil servants. Nevertheless, the most active third in the MRFIT group had a relative risk of CHD 20% below that of their least active cohort. The influence of physical activity in countering CHD was independent of other recognized predictors of that disease.

The bottom panel of Table 1 gives similar findings on 16,936 middle-aged male Harvard alumni followed for CHD incidence during 10 years (1962–1972) relative to their physical activity index in kilocalories per week assessed at entry (5,6). The alumni data included habitual walking and stair-climbing as well as leisure-time sportsplay activities self-assessed via mail questionnaires. About 40% of the alumni had a physical activity index of 2,000 kcal/week of leisure-time energy expenditure. In this group, 89% included some sportsplay in their habitual patterns, and 67% played vigorous sports, contrasted to only 30% and 20% with such sportsplaying among men with a lower index. The relative risk of CHD for the more active alumni was about 40% below that for the less active men.

Although the three studies cited in Table 1 differed considerably in their methodologies and populations, they show quite close parallels in their historical timing and their implications as to the inverse association of physical activity level and CHD risk. Both the British and the U.S. alumni studies demonstrated that vigorous sportsplay conferred additional benefits against CHD risk, over the protective influence attributed to moderate or nonvigorous physical activity. When the alumni follow-up was extended to 16 years, sportsplay of any sort was more beneficial than walking or stair-climbing without sports. The alumni study also held implications supporting remedial and interventional hypotheses, because college athletes lost CHD protection if they became inactive alumni, but graduates who had been less active as students acquired lower risk if they took up vigorous physical activity as alumni.

PHYSICAL FITNESS

Studies of physical fitness, measured primarily as cardiovascular or endurance fitness, have revealed important relationships to coronary artery health, and they point in the same direction as the physical activity findings just discussed. Fitness data (not tabulated here) from the MRFIT study (4) indicated that both treadmill time and the percentage of subjects achieving a target heart rate were significantly higher with increasing level of leisure-time physical activity, whereas resting and intermediate exercise heart rates were lower. The upper third of subjects by activity ratings had normal estimated mean functional capacity, while the least active group were below average in fitness. Accordingly, their levels of CHD risk were related inversely to their fitness status as well as to their physical activity status, and it has been postulated that the CHD benefits of exercise may be mediated in part by its influence on cardiovascular fitness.

Table 2 shows the findings of four epidemiological studies of physical fitness as related to CHD and all-cause mortality in Norwegian and American populations. The top panel presents data on 2,014 middle-aged male industrial and government workers in Oslo as classified by submaximal ergometer tests and followed for CHD mortality for 7 years (1975 to 1982) (7). When distributed into quartiles by increasing levels of fitness, the more fit men had lower blood pressure, lower heart rates, lower serum lipids, higher maximal heart rates and maximal blood pressures during exercise, and more favorable spirometry findings, than had those less fit. As seen in Table 2, physical fitness so assessed was a strong inverse predictor of fatal CHD in this population, with the risk in the most fit group reaching but one-fifth that of the least fit group.

The second panel of Table 2 shows relationships of all-cause mortality rates among 2,431 U.S. railway workers to their treadmill fitness test results (8). Exercise heart rates at various stages of testing were directly predictive of CHD death rates during the 20-year follow-up interval (1957–1977), with the rate corresponding to the slowest heart rate equaling but one-third of that corresponding to the fastest heart rate. The broad range of ages in this study population, together with its lengthy follow-up, add an impressive experience value to these observations. As in the MRFIT study, a high correlation was found between physical activity levels (both work and leisure-time) and ergometric fitness results (9).

Levels of fitness among 4,276 middle-aged men in a Lipid Research Clinics study were assessed by heart rate at stage 2 of a submaximal exercise test and

TABLE 2. *Relative risks of coronary heart disease (CHD) and all-cause mortality by levels of physical fitness in selected populations*

Norwegian industry and government workers[a]	Quartile of fitness by submaximal ergometry		CHD death rate per 100 men[e]	Relative risk of CHD death
7-yr follow-up, 1972–1982	1 (low)		5.7	1.00
	2		2.4	0.42
	3		2.2	0.39
	4 (high)		1.1	0.19
U.S. railway workers[b]	Exercise test heart rate	% of men	CHD death rate per 100 men[e]	Relative risk of CHD death
20-yr follow-up, 1957–1977	128+	22	13.2	1.00
	116–127	28	11.6	0.88
	106–115	27	8.7	0.66
	<106	23	9.1	0.69
Lipid research clinics subjects[c]	Quartile of fitness by submaximal ergometry		CHD death rate per 100 men[f]	Ratio of CHD death rate[g]
8.5-yr follow-up, 1972–1984	1 (low)		1.69	
	2		0.91	6.5
	3		0.91	(1.5–28.7)
	4 (high)		0.26	
Cooper Clinic subjects[d]	Quintile of fitness by maximal ergometry		All-cause death rate per 1,000 man–yr[f]	Ratio of all-cause death rate[h]
8-yr follow-up, 1972–1986	1 (low)		6.4	
	2		2.6	3.4
	3		2.7	(2.0–5.8)
	4		2.2	
	5 (high)		1.9	

[a] 2,014 men, ages 40 to 59 years at entry.
[b] 2,431 men, ages 22 to 79 years at entry.
[c] 4,276 men, ages 30 to 69 years at entry.
[d] 10,244 men, middle aged at entry.
[e] Adjusted for age differences; $p < 0.01$.
[f] Adjusted for age differences.
[g] Quartile 1:4 (95% CI).
[h] Quartile 1:5 (95% CI).

by time on treadmill (third panel, Table 2) (10). During an average 8.5-year follow-up (1972–1984), the cumulative CHD mortality among men in the least fit quartile was 6.5 times that of the most fit quartile. Adjustment for quartile differences in cigarette smoking, blood pressure level, and blood lipoprotein profile did not alter relative risks meaningfully. In fact, each of these adverse influences contributed independently to CHD mortality rates, as did physical fitness in its countering relationship.

The bottom panel of Table 2 summarizes the experience of 10,244 middle-aged men followed for 8 years (1972–1986) for their all-cause death rates as distributed by quintiles of fitness determined by maximal treadmill performance (11). Degree of fitness was based on age and sex norms of treadmill performance. Among these male executive and managerial clients of the Cooper Clinic in Dallas, Texas, mortality rates for the most fit were 70% lower than they were for the least fit quintile. Trends persisted after accounting for differences in cigarette-smoking habit; blood pressure, blood cholesterol, and blood glucose levels; and parental history of CHD. Similar but less dramatic differences were found among women tested at the Clinic.

LIFESTYLE AND LONGEVITY

Exercise, fitness, quality of living, and other elements of lifestyle have been considered for their relationships to all-cause mortality and longevity. All-cause death rates (not tabulated here) among the British civil servants during a 9-year follow-up were lower in men with an exercise-related reduction of CHD risk (1). Accordingly, their survival through middle-life into old age was greater than was survival among men who played no vigorous sports.

Table 3 shows relationships between physical activity and all-cause mortality in a group of 636 healthy middle-aged Finnish men between 1964 and 1984 (12), and among 16,936 Harvard alumni from 1962 to 1978 (13). These populations also were studied for estimated years of added life ascribed to favorable lifestyle characteristics. Of the Finnish men aged 45 to 64 years at entry, 287 died during the 20-year follow-up, 106 from CHD; however, men habitually vigorous during their daily activities lived an average of 2.1 years longer than

TABLE 3. *Relative risks of all-cause death by levels of physical activity in selected populations*

Finnish subjects[a]	Physical activity at baseline	No. men at baseline	Mean age at baseline	Mean age at death
20-yr follow-up, 1964–1984	Low	386	54.9	67.4
	High	250	55.2	69.1

Harvard alumni[b]	Physical activity index (kcal/wk)	Prevalence in man–yr (%)	All-cause death rate per 1,000 man–yr	Relative risk of all-cause death
16-yr follow-up, 1962–1978	<2,000	62	7.5	1.00
	2,000+	38	5.4	0.72

[a] 636 men, ages 45 to 64 years at entry; average added years of life from high activity = 2.1; adjusted for differences in age, blood pressure, serum cholesterol, and cigarette smoking; $p < 0.01$.

[b] 16,936 men, ages 35 to 74 years at entry; average added years of life to age 80 from high activity = 1.3; cigarette abstention = 2.3; and normotension = 2.7; adjusted for differences in age and each of other characteristics listed; $p < 0.01$ for each characteristic.

did those who were less active; the difference mainly because of their contrasting CHD mortality rates (top panel, Table 3). The saving was largely due to avoidance of premature death, and the survival curves for highly actives and low actives actually converged in the last 5 years of follow-up. This convergence of survival or death rates could have represented disappearance of differences in physical activity levels, altered influences of activity with aging, or the effect of some other attribute not assessed.

Of the college men aged 35 to 74 years at entry, 1,413 died during the 16-year follow-up, 441 from CHD. The more active men, who habitually expended more than 2,000 kcal/week in recreational physical activity, had a 28% lower risk of death from any cause during the follow-up than did their less active classmates (lower panel, Table 3). A gradient effect (not shown) indicated a steady decline in death rates as exercise levels increased from below 500 kcal/week to an optimum of 3,500. Actuarial models provided estimates of added years of life to be gained by having the benefit of an active way of life, as well as other favorable lifestyle elements. After adjusting for age and each of the other habits listed, the data suggest that the largest gain (2.7 years) would be achieved by avoiding hypertension; the second largest by not smoking cigarettes (2.3 years), and the third by being physically active enough to expend $\geq$2,000 kcal/week (1.3 years). A lifestyle combining all of these beneficial characteristics might be expected to gain further added life, since their influences are partly independent.

ACKNOWLEDGMENTS

This work was supported by U.S. Public Health Service Research Grant HL 34174 from the National Heart, Lung and Blood Institute.

REFERENCES

1. Morris JN, Everitt MG, Semmence AM. Exercise and coronary heart disease. In: Macleod D, Maughn R, Nimmo M, Reilly T, Williams C, eds. *Exercise: benefits, limits and adaptations.* London: E & FN Spon, 1987:4–19.
2. Morris JN. Physical activity in the prevention of cardiovascular disease. In: van Erp-Baart AMJ, Katan MB, Kemper HCG, van der Laan JAM, Morris JN, de Nobel E, Saris WHM, Weeds HWH, eds. *Inspanning en voeding,* Alphen aan den Rihn/Brussels: Samsom/Stafleu, 1985:54–63.
3. Morris JN. Exercise and the incidence of coronary heart disease. In: *Exercise–heart–health.* London: The Coronary Prevention Group, 1987:21–34.
4. Leon AS, Connett J, Jacobs DR Jr, Rauramaa R. Leisure-time physical activity levels and risk of coronary heart disease and death. The Multiple Risk Factor Intervention Trial. *JAMA* 1987;258:2388–2395.
5. Paffenbarger RS Jr, Wing AL, Hyde RT. Physical activity as an index of heart attack risk in college alumni. *Am J Epidemiol* 1978;108:161–175.
6. Paffenbarger RS Jr, Hyde RT, Wing AL, Steinmetz CH. A natural history of athleticism and cardiovascular health. *JAMA* 1984;252:491–495.

7. Lie H, Mundal R, Erikssen J. Coronary risk factors and incidence of coronary death in relation to physical fitness. Seven-year follow-up study of middle-aged and elderly men. *Eur Heart J* 1985;6:147–157.
8. Slattery ML, Jacobs DR. Physical fitness and cardiovascular disease mortality: The U.S. Railroad Study. *Am J Epidemiol* 1988;127:571–580.
9. Slattery ML, Jacobs DR Jr, Nichaman MZ. Leisure time physical activity and coronary heart disease death. The U.S. Railroad Study. *Circulation* 1989;79:304–311.
10. Ekelund L-G, Haskell WL, Johnson JL, Whaley FS, Criqui MH, Sheps DS. Physical fitness as a predictor of cardiovascular mortality in asymptomatic North American men. The Lipid Research Clinics mortality follow-up study. *N Engl J Med* 1988;319:1379–1384.
11. Blair SN, Kohl HW III, Paffenbarger RS Jr, Clark DG, Cooper KH, Gibbons LW. Physical fitness and all-cause mortality: A prospective study of healthy men and women. *JAMA* 1989;262:2395–2401.
12. Pekkanen J, Marti B, Nissinen A, Tuomilehto J. Reduction of premature mortality by high physical activity: A 20-year follow-up of middle-aged Finnish men. *Lancet* 1987;1:1473–1477.
13. Paffenbarger RS Jr, Hyde RT, Wing AL, Hsieh C-C. Physical activity, all cause-mortality, and longevity of college alumni. *N Engl J Med* 1986;314:605–613, and 315:399–401.

Atherosclerosis Reviews, Volume 21,
edited by A. Leaf and P. C. Weber.
Raven Press, Ltd., New York © 1990.

Alcohol Consumption and Its Relation to Hypertension and Coronary Heart Disease

Ulrich Keil

*Department of Social Medicine and Epidemiology, Ruhr-University Bochum,
Federal Republic of Germany*

A relationship between alcohol consumption and blood pressure (BP) elevation was first suggested by Lian in 1915, who noted that French servicemen drinking 2.5 liters of wine or more per day had increased prevalence of hypertension (1). Since 1967 attention has shifted to the question of whether an association exists between alcohol consumption and BP in populations not selected on the basis of alcohol intake. A large number of cross-sectional studies, a smaller number of prospective cohort studies, and a few experimental studies have addressed this question. Most studies have reported a positive association between alcohol consumption and BP (2).

Coronary heart disease (CHD) seems to be "the one condition most consistently suggesting that disease risk in moderate drinkers is lower than in nondrinkers" (3); a positive alcohol–CHD association has been seen only with higher amounts of alcohol consumption, thus producing a J-shaped or U-shaped curve for the alcohol–CHD relationship.

The following questions and topics of the alcohol–BP and alcohol–CHD relationship will be addressed in this article:

1. Difficulties in measuring alcohol consumption in population studies.
2. Is the alcohol–BP relationship linear, J-shaped, or U-shaped?
3. What are the major putative confounders of the alcohol–BP relationship?
4. Is there a threshold dose for hypertension risk?
5. What are the effects of modification of alcohol intake on BP?
6. What are the physiologic mechanisms for the alcohol–BP link?
7. Is the alcohol-CHD relationship linear, J-shaped, or U-shaped?
8. What are the major putative confounders of the alcohol–CHD relationship?
9. Is there a threshold dose for CHD risk?
10. What are the effects of modification of alcohol intake on CHD?
11. What are the physiologic mechanisms of the alcohol–CHD relationship?
12. To what extent does alcohol consumption contribute to the prevalence of hypertension and to the prevalence of CHD in the population?

13. How must epidemiological studies be improved to understand better the alcohol–BP and alcohol–CHD relationships?

MEASUREMENT PROBLEMS

Measurement of alcohol consumption is a fundamental issue in all population studies of the alcohol–BP relationship (3). One issue is the exact amount of alcohol consumed over a period such as a day, week, month or even longer periods. A second issue is the heterogeneity of the group that claims to consume no alcohol at all (3–5).

The blood-alcohol level usually is considered the "gold standard" for the amount of alcohol consumed. However, blood-alcohol determination becomes impractical when alcohol consumption in large numbers of people and over longer time periods must be assessed. Thus, in most epidemiologic studies investigators must rely on self reports of respondents. Self reports may be obtained by having participants keep daily diaries on their alcohol consumption. Another way is to recall consumption over periods ranging from the most recent week to the entire lifetime (3).

Studies on self-report measures generally indicate that heavy drinkers tend to underreport or even deny alcohol consumption (3,6,7). Also, it has been found that persons reporting to be teetotalers are often former heavy drinkers (3,5).

The "no-alcohol-consumption group" thus is a problem group comprising lifelong abstainers, former drinkers, drinkers who deny their alcohol consumption, and those who are too sick to drink alcohol. The separation of these subgroups who make up the "no-alcohol-consumption group" may alter the alcohol–BP and alcohol–CHD association (2,3).

It is likely that the above-mentioned misclassifications, especially among heavy drinkers and the "no-alcohol-consumption group," contribute to an underestimation of the strength of the alcohol–BP and alcohol–CHD association. It is also conceivable that the higher risk found for nondrinkers compared to low and moderate drinkers is an artifact. Furthermore, because of a general underreporting of alcohol consumption in most epidemiological studies, the estimation of a threshold dose might be too low (2,3).

EPIDEMIOLOGICAL AND EXPERIMENTAL STUDIES CONCERNING ALCOHOL AND HYPERTENSION

Cross-Sectional Studies

The alcohol–BP association has been investigated worldwide in at least 32 cross-sectional studies, 10 in Europe (2,8–17), 12 in North America (2,18–29), 6 in Australia (2,30–35), and 2 in New Zealand (36,37) and Japan (38,39) each.

All of the European studies found evidence of an alcohol–BP association independent of a number of putative confounding factors such as age, BMI, physical activity, smoking, coffee consumption, educational attainment, and Type A/B behavior. (Dietary intake was not assessed in most studies.)

In the Munich Blood Pressure Study (MBS) (12) and in the Lübeck Blood Pressure Study (LBS) (15), generally the BPs of nondrinkers were either greater than or no different from those of persons consuming 10 to 20 g of alcohol per day. In the LBS, BP was greater in drinkers than it was in nondrinkers at consumption levels of ≥40 g of alcohol per day. In the MBS, the respective alcohol consumption level was ≥60 g/day for men and ≥40 g/day for women.

The MONICA Augsburg Survey 1984/85 (17) confirmed the MBS results in that BP was clearly greater in drinkers than it was in nondrinkers at alcohol consumption levels of ≥60 g/day in men and ≥40 g/day in women. Among the three FRG studies performed with the same methodology, a clear J-shaped curve was found for the alcohol–SBP relationship (15) only in LBS men.

In the three FRG studies a strong interaction between alcohol consumption and smoking was found in older women (12,15); in the MONICA Augsburg Survey this interaction was found in men and women (17). Obviously, smoking can act as an effect modifier on the alcohol–BP relationship, i.e., Augsburg men who consume ≥60 g of alcohol per day and are smokers have 2 to 8 mm Hg higher systolic (SBP) and/or diastolic (DBP) BP values compared to nonsmokers. In LBS and MBS women ages 45 to 69 years this alcohol–smoking interaction was seen at alcohol levels ≥ 20 g/day. A physiological interpretation of this newly found interaction is not yet available (15).

With the exception of the Canada Health Study (26), all of the 12 North American studies have reported a statistically significant positive association of alcohol and BP. In the first Kaiser Permanente Study (20), only a small difference was found in SBPs or DBPs between nondrinking men and those consuming 10 to 20 g of alcohol per day. In women, SBPs and DBPs were greater in nondrinkers than they were in women consuming 10 to 20 g of alcohol per day. Thus, a J-shaped relationship was found in women. The findings of this study suggested that there might be a threshold effect of 30 g of alcohol per day for BP elevation in men and women and in all racial groups. Many more North American studies confirmed these findings (2,22,29).

With the exception of one study (31), the six Australian and the two New Zealand studies found linear, J-shaped and U-shaped associations between alcohol and BP. In the National Heart Foundation of Australia Risk Factor Prevalence Study (35) and in the Auckland Study (37) there was evidence of greater BP values in drinkers than in nondrinkers at consumption levels ≥ 30 g/day. Both Japanese studies (38,39) reported independent linear associations of alcohol with BP.

Prospective Cohort Studies

There are at least six prospective cohort studies of the alcohol-BP association (14,19,25,29,40,41). The results of all but the Honolulu Heart Study (41) are consistent with those of the cross-sectional studies and indicate a positive alcohol-BP association. The prospective association of alcohol with BP has been investigated over 4 years in the Framingham Study (25). In both men and women an increase in alcohol consumption over 4 years was associated with a significant increase in BP, whereas a decrease in alcohol consumption was associated with a significant decrease in BP.

Trials of Alcohol Restriction

Potter and Beevers (42) studied 16 men with hypertension whose alcohol consumption averaged 60 to 80 grams per day. They observed that BPs remained high when alcohol consumption was maintained at baseline levels but fell significantly (SBP 13 mm Hg; DBP 5 mm Hg) when alcohol was withdrawn for 3 to 4 days. When alcohol consumption was resumed significant increases in both SBP and DBP were observed.

The first randomized controlled trial of the effect of restriction of alcohol consumption on BP was carried out by Puddey et al. (43). These investigators studied 48 normotensive men who reported consuming an average of 40 to 50 g of alcohol per day in a 12-week cross-over trial; subjects consumed approximately 30 g of alcohol per day for 6 weeks and 30 g of alcohol per week for 6 weeks. Both SBPs and DBPs changed with reported changes in alcohol intake. The results of these studies suggest a short-term pressor effect of alcohol intake between 30 and 80 g/day in both hypertensive and normotensive subjects (2).

POSSIBLE MECHANISMS

The physiologic mechanisms by which long-term regular alcohol consumption leads to chronic elevations in BP are not yet clear. "The most attractive theory on present evidence to explain the mechanism of alcohol-induced hypertension is that of a direct effect of alcohol on vascular smooth muscle perhaps mediated by calcium influx" (44). There are indications that plasma calcium levels fall significantly after alcohol ingestion; to date it is not clear whether in the same subjects urinary calcium excretion is increased or not (45). At present neural, humoral, and renal mechanisms are discussed as mediators of the observed alcohol–BP association. The role of each of these factors, if any, is still unclear (2,46).

IMPLICATIONS FOR PREVENTION AND TREATMENT

In most epidemiological studies, BP levels were greater at alcohol consumption levels around ≥40 g/day than they were at levels of 10 to 20 g/day (2,15). About 25% of studies reported BP elevations at alcohol consumption levels < 30 g/day compared with BPs of nondrinkers (2). About 40% of studies reported BP of nondrinkers to be greater than BP of those consuming 10 to 20 g of alcohol per day (2). It is doubtful whether these findings actually reflect a BP-lowering effect of small amounts of alcohol. Thus, it is still unclear, whether the alcohol–BP relationship is linear or curvilinear. It is likely that the J-shaped relationship stems from the finding that "nondrinkers" are a heterogeneous group comprising extreme subgroups such as lifelong abstainers, heavy drinkers who deny their alcohol consumption, and those who are too ill to drink (3).

If a threshold dose for hypertension risk exists, it is probably around 30 to 60 g of alcohol per day (lower for women than for men).

From the public health perspective it is important to investigate what percentage of hypertension in the community might be caused by alcohol consumption and, more importantly, how much hypertension in the community could be eliminated if exposure to, e.g., ≥40 g of alcohol per day was eliminated. Focusing on the population-attributable-risk percent, it was calculated from LBS data that about 7% of hypertension in men in the community is due to alcohol consumption of ≥40 g/day (15). The respective calculations from U.S. and Australian population studies revealed that alcohol consumption could account for as much as 11% of hypertension in men but much less in women because of their much lesser alcohol consumption (35,47).

In spite of the many unanswered questions (e.g., threshold level and shape of the association) concerning the alcohol–BP relationship, it seems clear that a causal association exists between consumption of ≥30–60 g of alcohol per day and BP elevation in men and women. The statement of a causal relationship is justified because it has been shown that chance and, to a high degree, bias and confounding have been ruled out as possible explanations of the alcohol–BP association. It is most likely that the misclassifications of the exposure variable alcohol act in the direction of a dilution effect. Elimination of such misclassifications, therefore, should strengthen and not weaken the alcohol–BP association. Furthermore, the consistency of the cross-sectional, prospective cohort and experimental studies is high. In addition, the request for a clear-time sequence between cause and effect has been fulfilled. However, the request for biological plausibility must be pursued further.

Interestingly enough, alcohol consumption ≥ 30–60 g/day is seen today to be the second most important risk factor for hypertension, closely behind the well-established risk factor of being overweight.

EPIDEMIOLOGICAL AND EXPERIMENTAL STUDIES CONCERNING ALCOHOL AND CORONARY HEART DISEASE

When considering the alcohol–CHD association one must distinguish between two separate issues: the harmful effect of heavy drinking and the effect of light to moderate drinking, which might be harmless or even beneficial (48,49).

Studies on Alcoholics and Problem Drinkers

At least seven mortality studies of alcoholics and problem drinkers have been reported (48,49). In each of these studies the relative risk for heavy drinking was statistically significantly >1.0 (relative risk between 1.2 and 3.6.) (48).

Ecological Studies

International ecological studies based on aggregate data have found an inverse relationship between per capita alcohol consumption and CHD mortality rates in many countries (48).

Case-Control and Prospective Cohort Studies

Many case control studies consistently have shown less risk of CHD in low to moderate alcohol users compared to nonusers (48). Cohort studies specifically designed to study CHD have shown the same associations seen in case-control studies (3,48,50). Among these studies the Chicago Western Electric Study is an exception in that persons reporting alcohol consumption $\geq$ 60 g/day had increased CHD mortality compared to nondrinkers (51).

Experimental Studies

Because of ethical reasons experimental studies have been done only on nonhuman primates. Autopsies on monkeys "fed a high cholesterol diet showed that those randomly assigned to alcohol had only 8% of their arteries stenosed with plaque, whereas those assigned to the alcohol placebo group had 48% of their arteries stenosed" (49).

Comments

It is conceivable that in many case-control and prospective cohort studies heavy alcohol users were misclassified into light and moderate consumer categories; such a misclassification can alter study findings considerably (3,52). Also, it is conceivable that the effects of putative confounders such as income and educational attainment on CHD morbidity and mortality have not been controlled for sufficiently in many studies (3). It has been shown that lifelong abstainers have lower levels of education and income compared to persons who consume alcohol (53,54). Thus, the higher mortality found among teetotalers as compared to moderate drinkers may reflect their lower socioeconomic status (3).

Studies suggesting alcohol to be harmful tend to show this at moderate to high levels; CHD death tends to be the outcome variable of these studies (49).

The evidence that alcohol is protective for CHD at low doses is still inconsistent (49,60). In light of the inconsistent findings from epidemiological studies concerning the effect of light to moderate consumption of alcohol on CHD, an understanding of the possible mechanisms by which alcohol may exert a beneficial effect on CHD is of great importance (3,48,49).

POSSIBLE MECHANISMS

Alcohol intake elevates HDL-cholesterol. This physiologic effect of alcohol supports the view of a protective effect of low to moderate alcohol use on CHD risk (48,49,55). Another mechanism by which moderate alcohol consumption might protect against CHD is an inhibition of platelet aggregation (48). Alcohol also potentiates the antiplatelet effect of aspirin (56). Alcohol-induced thrombocytopenia has been described (57) also. However, if we see the alcohol–BP association as a linear relationship, this association does not help to explain a possibly protective effect of moderate alcohol consumption on CHD.

Increased alcohol consumption could lead to increased fibrinolytic activity, and along with the platelet effects these could be additional mechanisms "explaining" a protective effect of alcohol (49,58,61).

To understand better the basic mechanisms of the alcohol–CHD association, it is important to examine the alcohol–CHD relationship in the context of all other CHD risk factors, especially in the context of overall dietary intakes. It is still conceivable that the type of dietary difference between alcohol consumption categories rather than alcohol consumption itself is what reduces the risk of CHD (48).

IMPLICATIONS FOR PREVENTION AND TREATMENT

The alcohol–CHD association must be viewed in a broader public health perspective. Any possibly beneficial effects of the prescription of moderate amounts of alcohol must be considered in the context that alcohol consumption is implicated in 25% of all general hospital admissions, in 40% of all deaths from traffic accidents, and in 50% of all criminal arrests (48). A major public health question reads as follows: Is the level of alcohol consumption that possibly protects against CHD harmful with regard to other major diseases? In addition, the following point must be considered: Chronic alcohol use has a toxic effect on the myocardium, thus impairing ventricular performance (49).

Until the relationship between alcohol consumption, other CHD risk factors such as diet, and CHD have been explored in more depth, alcohol should not be prescribed to prevent CHD. To date there are too many unanswered questions to make any public health recommendations concerning the intake of moderate amounts of alcohol as a way to prevent CHD (3,48,49).

"A randomized trial of alcohol dosing would probably be the best way to assess the ratio of long-term risks to benefits" (49). However, because of ethical reasons such a trial can hardly ever be performed.

CONCLUSIONS AND RECOMMENDATIONS

From all epidemiological studies investigating the alcohol–BP and the alcohol–CHD associations, it has become clear that the accurate assessment of alcohol consumption is the paramount and crucial problem (2,3,48,49). Addressing this problem, Colsher and Wallace (3) have made the following recommendations:

1. "In analyzing the current alcohol nonuser category, separate prior users from lifelong abstainers. Where possible obtain measures that may inform as to the heterogeneity of alcohol-use categories.
2. "If at all possible screen all study participants for an alcohol abuse and alcoholism history with an instrument such as the Michigan Alcoholism Screening Test (59) to help reduce misclassification of alcohol use.
3. "Construct alcohol use items to reflect more accurately drinking patterns, especially in moderate to heavy occasional use.
4. "Separately record alcohol intake in the 24 to 48 hr prior to study if alcohol-related physiologic or biochemical measures are to be obtained." (4)

It is conceivable that a major improvement in the assessment of the exposure variable alcohol will contribute to a stronger alcohol–BP and alcohol–CHD association and will transform the frequently found J-shaped curves to a more linear relationship with a threshold dose of approximately 30 to 60 g of alcohol per day for hypertension and a possibly higher threshold for CHD.

ACKNOWLEDGMENTS

The preparation of the manuscript by Carmen Ewe is gratefully acknowledged.

REFERENCES

1. Lian C. L'alcoholisme, cause d'hypertension arterielle. *Bull Acad Natl Med (Paris)* 1915;74: 525–528.
2. MacMahon S. Alcohol consumption and hypertension. *Hypertension* 1987;9:111–121.
3. Colsher PL, Wallace RB. Is modest alcohol consumption better than none at all? An epidemiologic assessment. *Annu Rev Public Health* 1989;10:203–219.
4. Ferrence RA, Truscott S, Whitehead PC. Drinking and the prevention of coronary heart disease: findings, issues, and public health policy. *J Stud Alcohol* 1986;47:394–408.
5. Knupfer G. Drinking for health: the daily light drinker myth. *Br J Addict* 1987;82:547–555.
6. Chick J. Epidemiology of alcohol use and its hazards, with a note on screening methods. *Br Med Bull* 1982;38:3–8.
7. Poikolainen K, Karkkainen P. Diary gives more accurate information about alcohol consumption than questionnaire. *Drug Alcohol Depend* 1983;11:209–216.

8. Gyntelberg F, Meyer J. Relationship between blood pressure and physical fitness, smoking and alcohol consumption in Copenhagen males aged 40–59. *Acta Med Scand* 1974;195:375–380.
9. Kozararevic DJ, Vojvodic N, Dawber T. Frequency of alcohol consumption and morbidity and mortality: the Yugoslavia Cardiovascular Disease Study. *Lancet* 1980;1:613–616.
10. Milon H, Froment A, Gaspard P, Guidollet J, Ripole JP. Alcohol consumption and blood pressure in a French epidemiological study. *Eur Heart J* 1982;3:59–64.
11. Salonen JT, Tuomilehto J, Tanskanen A. Relation of blood pressure to reported intake of salt, saturated fats, and alcohol in a healthy middle aged population. *J Epidemiol Community Health* 1983;37:32–37.
12. Cairns V, Keil U, Kleinbaum D, Doering A, Stieber J. Alcohol consumption as a risk factor for high blood pressure: Munich Blood Pressure Study. *Hypertension* 1984;6:124–131.
13. Kornhuber HH, Lisson G, Suschka-Sauermann L. Alcohol and obesity: a new look at high blood pressure and stroke; an epidemiological study in preventive neurology. *Eur Arch Psychiatry Neurol Sci* 1985;234:357–362.
14. Kromhout D, Bosschieter EB, Coulander CL. Potassium, calcium, alcohol intake and blood pressure: the Zutphen Study. *Am J Clin Nutr* 1985;41:1299–1304.
15. Keil U, Chambless L, Remmers A. Alcohol and blood pressure: results from the Lübeck Blood Pressure Study. *Prev Med* 1989;18:1–10.
16. Bulpitt CJ, Shipley MJ, Semmence A. The contribution of a moderate intake of alcohol to the presence of hypertension. *J Hypertens* 1987;5:85–91.
17. Keil U, Chambless L, Filipiak B, Härtel U. Alcohol and blood pressure and its interaction with smoking and other behavioural variables: results from the MONICA Augsburg Survey 1984/ 85. (Submitted.)
18. Clark VA, Chapman JM, Coulson AH. Effects of various factors on systolic and diastolic blood pressure in the Los Angeles Heart Study. *J Chronic Dis* 1967;20:571–581.
19. Dyer AR, Stamler J, Paul O. Alcohol consumption, cardiovascular risk factors and mortality in two Chicago epidemiologic studies. *Circulation* 1977;56:1067–1074.
20. Klatsky AL, Friedman GD, Siegeland AB, Gerard MJ. Alcohol consumption and blood pressure. *N Engl J Med* 1977;296:1194–1200.
21. Harburg E, Ozgoren F, Hawthorne VM, Schork MA. Community norms of alcohol usage and blood pressure. *Am J Public Health* 1980;70:813–820.
22. Criqui MH, Wallace RB, Mishkel M, Barrett-Conner E, Heiss G. Alcohol consumption and blood pressure: the Lipid Research Clinics Prevalence Study. *Hypertension* 1981;3:557–565.
23. Kagan A, Yano K, Rhoads GG, McGee DL. Alcohol and cardiovascular disease: the Hawaiian experience. *Circulation* 1981;64(suppl 3):27–31.
24. Fortmann SP, Haskell WL, Vranizan K, Brown BW, Farquhar JW. The association of blood pressure and dietary alcohol: differences by age, sex and estrogen use. *Am J Epidemiol* 1983;118:497–507.
25. Gordon T, Kannel WB. Drinking and its relation to smoking, blood pressure, blood lipids and uric acid. *Arch Intern Med* 1983;143:1366–1374.
26. Coates RA, Corey PN, Ashley MJ, Steele CA. Alcohol consumption and blood pressure: analysis of data from the Canada Health Survey. *Prev Med* 1985;14:1–14.
27. Gruchow HW, Sobocinski KA, Barboriak JJ. Alcohol, nutrient intake, and hypertension in US adults. *JAMA* 1985;253:1567–1570.
28. Klatsky AL, Friedman GD, Armstrong MA. The relationships between alcoholic beverage use and other traits to blood pressure: a new Kaiser Permanente study. *Circulation* 1986;73:628–636.
29. Gordon T, Doyle JT. Alcohol consumption and its relationship to smoking, weight, blood pressure, and blood lipids: the Albany Study. *Arch Intern Med* 1986;146:262–265.
30. Mitchell PI, Morgan MJ, Boadle DJ. The role of alcohol in the etiology of hypertension. *Med J Aust* 1980;2:198–200.
31. Baghurst K, Dwyer T. Alcohol consumption and blood pressure in a group of young Australian males. *J Human Nutr* 1981;35:257–264.
32. Cooke KM, Frost GW, Thornell IR, Stokes GS. Alcohol consumption and blood pressure: survey of the relationship in a health screening clinic. *Med J Aust* 1982;1:65–69.
33. Arkwright PD, Beilin LJ, Rouse I, Armstrong BK, Vandongen R. Effects of alcohol use and other aspects of lifestyle on blood pressure levels and the prevalence of hypertension in a working population. *Circulation* 1982;66:60–66.

34. Savdie E, Grosslight GM, Adena MA. Relation of alcohol and cigarette consumption to blood pressure and serum creatinine levels. *J Chronic Dis* 1984;37:617–623.
35. MacMahon SW, Blacket RB, MacDonald GJ, Hall W. Obesity, alcohol consumption and blood pressure in Australian men and women. The National Heart Foundation of Australia Risk Factor Prevalence Study. *J Hypertens* 1984;2:85–91.
36. Paulin JM, Simpson FO, Waal-Manning HJ. Alcohol consumption and blood pressure in a New Zealand community study. *NZ Med J* 1985;98:425–428.
37. Jackson R, Stewart A, Beaglehole R, Scragg R. Alcohol consumption and blood pressure. *Am J Epidemiol* 1985;122:1034–1044.
38. Ueshima H, Shimamoto T, Iada M. Alcohol intake and hypertension among urban and rural Japanese populations. *J Chronic Dis* 1984;37:585–592.
39. Kondo K, Ebihara A. Alcohol consumption and blood pressure in a rural community of Japan: In: Lovenberg W, Yamori Y, eds. *Nutritional prevention of cardiovascular disease.* Orlando, FL: Academic Press. 1984:217–224.
40. Dyer AR, Stamler J, Paul O. Alcohol, cardiovascular risk factors and mortality: The Chicago experience. *Circulation* 1981;64(suppl 3):20–27.
41. Reed D, McGee D, Katsuhiko Y. Biological and social correlates of blood pressure among Japanese men in Hawaii. *Hypertension* 1982;4:406–414.
42. Potter JF, Beevers DG. Pressor effect of alcohol in hypertension. *Lancet* 1984;1:119–122.
43. Puddey IB, Beilin LJ, Vandongen R, Rouse IR, Rogers P. Evidence for a direct effect of alcohol consumption on blood pressure in normotensive men: a randomized controlled trial. *Hypertension* 1985;7:707–713.
44. Maheswaran R, Potter JF, Beevers DG. The role of alcohol in hypertension. *J Clin Hypertens* 1986;2:172–178.
45. Potter JF, Watson RDS, Skan W, Beevers DG. The pressor and metabolic effects of alcohol in normotensive subjects. *Hypertension* 1986;8:625–631.
46. Klatsky AL. Blood pressure and alcohol intake. In: *Hypertension: pathophysiology, diagnosis, and management.* Laragh JH, Brenner BM, eds. New York: Raven Press. 1990:277–294.
47. Friedman GD, Klatsky AL, Siegelaub AB. Alcohol, tobacco and hypertension. *Hypertension* 1982;4(suppl 3):143–150.
48. Hennekens CH. Alcohol. In: Kaplan NM, Stamler J, eds. *Prevention of coronary heart disease. Practical management of the risk factors.* Philadelphia: WB Saunders. 1983:130–138.
49. Fraser GE. *Preventive cardiology.* 1st ed. New York: Oxford University Press, 1986:184–194.
50. Moore RD, Pearson TA. Moderate alcohol consumption and coronary heart disease. A review. *Medicine* 1986;65:242–267.
51. Dyer AR, Stamler J, Paul O. Alcohol consumption and 17 year mortality in the Chicago Western Electric Company Study. *Prev Med* 1980;9:78–90.
52. Blackwelder WC, Yano K, Rhoads GG. Alcohol and mortality: The Honolulu Heart Study. *Am J Med* 1980;68:164–169.
53. Goodwin DW, Johnson J, Maher C, Rappaport A, Guze SB. Why people do not drink: a study of teetotalers. *Compr Psychiatry* 1969;10:209–214.
54. Wallace JG. Drinkers and abstainers in Norway. A national survey. *Q J Studies Alcohol* 1972;33(suppl 6):129–151.
55. Castelli WP, Gordon T, Hjortland MC. Alcohol and blood lipids. *Lancet* 1977;2:153.
56. Deykin D, Janson P, McMahon L. Ethanol potentiation of aspirin induced prolongation of the bleeding time. *N Engl J Med* 1982;306:852–854.
57. Haut MJ, Cowan DH. The effect of ethanol on hemostatic properties of human blood platelets. *Am J Med* 1974;56:22–23.
58. Meade TW, Chakrabarti R, Haines AP. Characteristics affecting fibrinolytic activity and plasma fibrinogen concentrations. *Br Med J* 1979;1:153.
59. Selzer ML. The Michigan Alcoholism Screening Test: the quest for a new diagnostic instrument. *Am J Psychiatry* 1971;127:469–472.
60. Shaper AG, Wannamethee G, Walker M. Alcohol and mortality in British men: explaining the U-shaped curve. *Lancet* 1988;2:1267–73.
61. Criqui MH. The roles of alcohol in the epidemiology of cardiovascular diseases. *Acta Med Scand* 1987;suppl 717:73–85.

Atherosclerosis Reviews, Volume 21,
edited by A. Leaf and P. C. Weber.
Raven Press, Ltd., New York © 1990.

Cellular Interactions, Growth Factors, and Atherogenesis

Russell Ross

Department of Pathology, University of Washington, Seattle, Washington 98195

The lesions of atherosclerosis range from the ubiquitous fatty streak, which consists largely of lipid-laden, monocyte-derived macrophages intermixed with varying numbers of T-lymphocytes, to the semiocclusive, smooth-muscle-proliferative lesion, sometimes called the fibrous plaque or complicated lesion (1,2). The fibrous plaque consists of a complicated cellular lesion that is covered by a fibrous cap of dense connective tissue consisting of smooth muscle cells sitting in lacunar-like spaces, surrounded by a dense connective tissue matrix, and intermixed with varying numbers of macrophages (3,4). This fibrous cap covers a deeper layer of macrophages, many of which contain lipid and appear as foam cells, together with varying amounts of cell debris, necrotic material, and extracellular lipid. Beneath this area of central necrosis, there is often a region of proliferated smooth muscle cells and connective tissue. The fibrous plaque often undergoes further changes in which the surface becomes ulcerated or the lesion becomes cracked or fissured. When this occurs, mural thrombi may form at the surface. Such thrombosis may lead to occlusive thrombi and the ultimate clinical sequelae of infarction, gangrene, or loss of extremity function. The complicated and advanced lesions of atherosclerosis contain four cell types: monocyte-derived macrophages; T-lymphocytes (both CD-8- and CD-4-positive cells); endothelial cells, particularly in vascularized lesions that contain vasa vasorum; and large numbers of proliferated smooth muscle cells. It is the smooth muscle proliferation that determines whether or not a lesion progresses from a fatty streak to a fibrous plaque that can occlude a given artery (1,2).

LESION PROGRESSION

As the fatty streak progresses to a fibrous plaque, it undergoes a series of intermediate changes involving both smooth muscle migration and proliferation. On some occasions, fatty streaks may form in loci (principally near branches and bifurcations) in the vessel wall where preexisting accumulations of intimal smooth muscle cells occur on a developmental basis. These intimal accumulations are sometimes called cushions. In other anatomic loci, the fatty streak appears to form at sites that subsequently become intermixed with smooth muscle cells, which appear to have migrated from the underlying media of the artery into the intima, where many of them go on to proliferate and create a mixed macrophage/smooth muscle/T-cell-containing lesion (5). This fibrofatty, or intermediate, lesion may become complicated further and with time can develop into a fibrous plaque or complicated lesion. The intimal proliferation of smooth muscle cells lies at the heart of the changes that occur during the progression of the fatty streak to a fibrous plaque. Therefore, understanding the basis of this proliferation may provide clues to means of intervening and preventing the formation of the occlusive lesions of atherosclerosis.

THE ROLE OF THE MACROPHAGE

Because the macrophage is ubiquitous in all lesions of atherosclerosis, together with varying numbers of T-lymphocytes, it has been suggested that an immune or autoimmune response may be involved, in some cases at least, in the process of atherogenesis (6). Interactions among T-lymphocytes and macrophages may be important components of macrophage activation, although it is not yet known what kinds of cytokines and growth-regulatory molecules may be formed and secreted by these two cell types as they interact. Macrophages have been known for some time to be a source of growth factors (7), and recently have been demonstrated to be a rich source of platelet-derived growth factor (PDGF) (8,9). They also can provide growth-regulatory molecules that include interleukin-1 (IL-1) (10), transforming growth factor-beta (TGFβ) (11), tumor necrosis factor-alpha (TNFα) (12), as well as numerous other growth-regulatory molecules. Since macrophages, smooth muscle, and endothelium all can present antigens, they also may be involved in immune-complex formation, should it occur within the artery wall. Because of their ability to form PDGF A- and B-chains, it has been suggested that macrophages might play a critical role in both the chemotactic and proliferative smooth muscle events seen during lesion progression (13).

SMOOTH MUSCLE CELLS

Smooth muscle cells are not only responsible for the proliferative events that occur during lesion progression, but they are also the key cells involved in the formation of the connective tissue matrix that comprises the lesion. In fact, many lesions of atherosclerosis are highly fibrous, whereas others may be very rich in lipid and are relatively nonfibrous. This will vary from patient to patient and is associated with the genetic makeup of individuals and the levels of risk factors to which they are exposed. Smooth muscle cells, which contain both types of PDGF receptors (α and β receptors), recently have been demonstrated to be capable also of forming endogenous PDGF-AA after stimulation with molecules such as IL-1 (14). Thus, in some circumstances, smooth muscle cells within the artery may be capable of autocrine stimulation in the appropriate local microenvironment (14).

PLATELET-DERIVED GROWTH FACTOR (PDGF)

Platelet-derived growth factor is one of the more important candidates for the molecule responsible for the intimal smooth-muscle-proliferative response. The basis for this assumption is that PDGF is present in platelets and can be formed by endothelium, smooth muscle, and macrophages, all of which may be activated to synthesize and secrete PDGF in the microenvironment of the arterial intima (15).

PDGF consists of a dimer of the A-chain and the B-chain, which are 60% homologous with each other. Three dimeric forms (AA, BB, AB) are found in platelets, and one or more of them can be formed by each of the cells within the artery wall. Susceptible cells such as smooth muscle contain two receptor subunits (termed α and β). Different cell types contain varying ratios of these receptor subunits. The mature PDGF receptor is formed by two of the subunits within the plane of the cell plasma membrane that come together to bind to the covalently bound dimeric form of PDGF. The α PDGF receptor subunit can bind to either the A- or the B-chain of PDGF, whereas the β subunit can bind to only the B-chain. Therefore, the ratio of α to β subunits presented by a given cell type is critical in determining the relative susceptibility of each cell to the mitogenic activity of the specific dimeric form of PDGF (16,17). For example, cells such as human dermal fibroblasts contain a 20:1 ratio of β:α receptors. In these circumstances, PDGF-BB is a very potent mitogen for fibroblasts, whereas PDGF-AA is a relatively poor mitogen for these cells. In contrast, 3T3 cells and some strains of smooth muscle cells contain 1:1 or 2:1 ratios of β:α subunits. In these circumstances, PDGF-AA, -BB, and -AB are equally potent mitogens for such cells. It becomes critical, therefore, to determine the relative numbers of PDGF receptor subunits, as well as to have knowledge of the dimeric form of PDGF to which the cells will be exposed, if one is to know how potentially mitogenic the available form of PDGF may be in these circumstances.

CELLULAR INTERACTIONS

In studies of nonhuman primates (18–21), which have been corroborated recently in studies of human hearts that have been removed to be replaced by transplants (22), it has been demonstrated that the first cellular interactions that occur in hyperlipidemic individuals consist of adhesion of monocytes and lymphocytes at branch points and bifurcations in the arterial tree, where the blood flow is slowed and eddy currents and back currents form. The monocytes then can be seen to migrate between endothelial cells and to locate subendo-thelially, where they may become activated as macrophages and may take up lipid and appear as foam cells. Thus, fatty streaks are formed. With time, these lesions may increase in size by continuing recruitment of monocytes and lymphocytes. Eventually, smooth muscle cells appear intermixed between and among the aggregated monocyte/macrophages and T-lymphocytes. At some point, many of the foam cells, which represent macrophages that have accumulated large amounts of lipid in the form of cholesterol and cholesterol esters, may break through the surface of the endothelium by inducing separation of the endothelial junctions, where they once again become exposed to the blood flow. At such sites, mural thrombi may form on the exposed macrophage surfaces. In these regions, it is not uncommon to find what appears to be a fairly rapid formation of smooth-muscle-proliferative lesions. It has been suggested that both the platelet aggregates and the cells within the artery wall may be responsible for the growth-regulatory molecules that lead to the intimal proliferative-smooth-muscle response. PDGF is one of the prime candidates for this response. In this regard, it has been demonstrated recently that nonlipid-containing macrophages in all of the observed lesions of human atherosclerosis as well as nonhuman primate atherosclerosis contain PDGF-BB and/or PDGF-AB protein (23). This has been observed by using a monoclonal antibody that is specific for the B-chain of PDGF, which recognizes PDGF-BB and PDGF-AB but not PDGF-AA. Using this monoclonal antibody together with monoclonal antibodies that recognize cell specificity, double immunohistochemical staining of the lesions of atherosclerosis demonstrates the presence of PDGF-B-chain–containing protein within numerous nonfoam-cell macrophages in the lesions. Thus, for the first time it can be demonstrated that the macrophage is clearly a source of PDGF during the process of atherogenesis.

RESPONSE-TO-INJURY HYPOTHESIS

The response-to-injury hypothesis of atherosclerosis originally postulated that some form of endothelial dysfunction leads to leukocyte interactions and the subendothelial localization of these leukocytes associated with intimal migration and/or proliferation of smooth muscle cells, which eventually culminates in the genesis of atherosclerotic lesions (Fig. 1). Furthermore, it has been suggested that the dysfunction of the endothelium permits a number of events that lead to activation of monocyte/macrophages and altered metabolism of smooth muscle cells, T-lymphocytes, and possibly endothelial cells, leading to the generation of growth-regulatory molecules such as PDGF. This hypothesis, which has continued to be modified over the years, has provided a framework in which numerous questions may be addressed concerning the control of the cellular interactions and the natures of the molecules they release. It has been valuable in permitting further experimentation and the design of future tools that may help us to develop better diagnosis and treatment approaches as well as new methods of prevention.

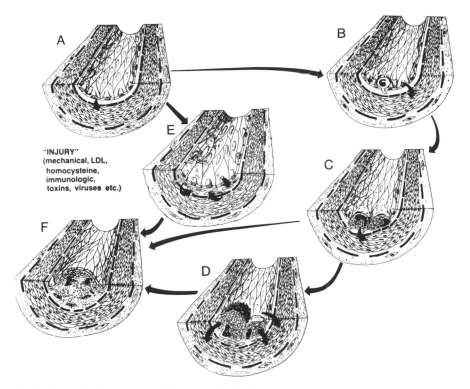

FIG. 1. The revised response-to-injury hypothesis. Advanced intimal proliferative lesions of atherosclerosis may occur by at least two pathways. The pathway demonstrated by the clockwise (long) arrows to the right has been observed in experimentally induced hypercholesterolemia. Injury to the endothelium (A) may induce growth factor secretion (short arrow). Monocytes attach to endothelium (B), which may continue to secrete growth factors (short arrow). Subendothelial migration of monocytes (C) may lead to fatty-streak formation and release of growth factors such as PDGF (short arrow). Fatty streaks may become converted directly to fibrous plaques (long arrow from C to F) through release of growth factors from macrophages or endothelial cells or both. Macrophages also may stimulate or injure the overlying endothelium. In some cases, macrophages may lose their endothelial cover and platelet attachment may occur (D), providing three possible sources of growth factors—platelets, macrophages, and endothelium (short arrows). Some of the smooth-muscle cells in the proliferative lesion itself (F) may form and secrete growth factors such as PDGF (short arrows). An alternative pathway for development of advanced lesions of atherosclerosis is shown by the arrows from A to E to F. In this case, the endothelium may be injured but remain intact. Increased endothelial turnover may result in growth-factor formation by endothelial cells (A). This may stimulate migration of smooth-muscle cells from the media into the intima, accompanied by endogenous production of PDGF by smooth muscle as well as growth-factor secretion from the "injured" endothelial cells (E). These interactions could lead then to fibrous-plaque formation and further lesion progression (F). From ref. 13.

ACKNOWLEDGMENTS

This work was supported in part by NIH grant HL-18645 to RR, NIH grant RR-00166 to the Northwest Regional Primate Center, and NIH grant HL-03174-33 to S. Schwartz.

REFERENCES

1. Ross R, Glomset JA. Atherosclerosis and the arterial smooth muscle cell. *Science* 1973;180: 1332–1339.
2. Ross R, Glomset JA. The pathogenesis of atherosclerosis. *N Engl J Med* 1976;295:369–377, 420–425.
3. Ross R, Wight TN, Strandness E, Thiele B. Human atherosclerosis. I. Cell constitution and characteristics of advanced lesions of the superficial femoral artery. *Am J Pathol* 1984;114:79–93.
4. Gown AM, Tsukada T, Ross R. Human atherosclerosis. II. Immunocytochemical analysis of the cellular composition of human atherosclerotic lesions. *Am J Pathol* 1986;125:191–207.
5. Stary HC. Macrophages, macrophage foam cells, and eccentric thickening in the coronary arteries of young children. *Atherosclerosis* 1987;64:91–108.
6. Hansson GK, Jonasson L, Seifert PS, Stemme S. Immune mechanisms in atherosclerosis. *Arteriosclerosis* 1989;9:567–579.
7. Leibovich SJ, Ross R. A macrophage-dependent factor that stimulates the proliferation of fibroblasts *in vitro. Am J Pathol* 1976;84:501–513.
8. Glenn KC, Ross R. Human monocyte-derived growth factor(s) for mesenchymal cells: activation of secretion by endotoxin and Concanavalin A. *Cell* 1981;25:603–615.
9. Shimokado K, Raines EW, Madtes DK, Barrett TB, Benditt EP, Ross R. A significant part of macrophage-derived growth factor consists of at least two forms of PDGF. *Cell* 1985;43:277–286.
10. Dinarello CA. Interleukin-1. *Rev Infect Dis* 1984;6:51–95.
11. Assoian RK, Fleurdelys BE, Stevenson HC, et al. Expression and secretion of type β transforming growth factor by activated human macrophages. *Proc Natl Acad Sci USA* 1987;84:6020–6024.
12. Nathan CF. Secretory products of macrophages. *J Clin Invest* 1987;79:319–26.
13. Ross R. The pathogenesis of atherosclerosis—an update. *N Engl J Med* 1986;314:488–500.
14. Raines EW, Dower SK, Ross R. IL-1 mitogenic activity for fibroblasts and smooth muscle cells is due to PDGF-AA. *Science* 1989;243:393–396.
15. Ross R, Raines EW, Bowen-Pope DF. The biology of platelet-derived growth factor. *Cell* 1986;46:155–169.
16. Seifert RA, Hart CE, Phillips PE, Forstrom JW, Ross R, Murray MJ, Bowen-Pope DF. Two different subunits associate to create isoform-specific platelet-derived growth factor receptors. *J Biol Chem* 1989;264:8771–8778.
17. Heldin C-H, Backstrom G, Ostman A, et al. Binding of different dimeric forms of PDGF to human fibroblasts: evidence for two separate receptor types. *EMBO J* 1988;7:1387–1393.
18. Faggiotto A, Ross R, Harker L. Studies of hypercholesterolemia in the nonhuman primate. I. Changes that lead to fatty streak formation. *Arteriosclerosis* 1984;4:323–340.
19. Faggiotto A, Ross R. Studies of hypercholesterolemia in the nonhuman primate. II. Fatty streak conversion to fibrous plaque. *Arteriosclerosis* 1984;4:341–356.
20. Masuda J, Ross R. Atherogenesis during low-level hypercholesterolemia in the nonhuman primate. I. Fatty streak formation. *Arteriosclerosis* 1990;10:164–177.
21. Masuda J, Ross R. Atherogenesis during low-level hypercholesterolemia in the nonhuman primate. II. Fatty streak conversion to fibrous plaque. *Arteriosclerosis* 1990;10:178–187.
22. Davies MJ, Woolf N, Rowles PM, Pepper J. Morphology of the endothelium over atherosclerotic plaques in human coronary arteries. *Br Heart J* 1988;60:459–464.
23. Ross R, Masuda J, Raines EW, et al. Localization of PDGF-B protein in macrophages in all phases of atherogenesis. *Science* (in press).

Atherosclerosis Reviews, Volume 21,
edited by A. Leaf and P. C. Weber.
Raven Press, Ltd., New York © 1990.

The Role of Monocytes and Oxidized LDL in Atherosclerosis

Joseph L. Witztum

*Department of Medicine, University of California,
San Diego, La Jolla, California 92093*

Atherosclerosis is a multifactorial disease involving a complex array of circulating blood proteins, lipoproteins and cells, and their interactions with the cells and matrix proteins of the arterial wall. The end-stage lesion, which leads to the occlusion of a vessel, or provides the thrombogenic surface for the initiation of a potentially fatal intravascular thrombosis, is in large part an acellular, fibrotic section of tissue containing the cellular debris of generations of dead and decaying cells and a variety of substances trapped amidst this debris. Prominent among these materials is cholesterol, chiefly in the form of precipitated crystals (1).

THE ATHEROSCLEROTIC PLAQUE

Although many pathogenic mechanisms must be involved in transforming normal arterial tissue to this end stage, it is clear that deposition of cholesterol within the arterial wall plays a central role in the pathogenesis of the atherosclerotic plaque. Because the cholesterol of the arterial wall is derived from circulative lipoproteins, chiefly in the form of low-density lipoproteins (LDL), any scheme that seeks to describe the sequence of events that results in plaque must take into account the mechanism(s) by which LDL accumulates (2–4). Thus, the "lipid hypothesis" does not state that an elevation of LDL is the only cause of atherogenesis—quite the contrary, as it is apparent that the etiology is multifactorial. However, the lipid hypothesis does state that circulating cholesterol (principally in the form of LDL) is central to the atherogenic process and that without "sufficient" plasma levels atherogenesis cannot proceed (2,5).

The advanced plaque, as noted above, is in large part acellular, fibrotic, and has grossly distorted arterial wall architecture and vasomotor function. Therapies designed at reversing this complex lesion are less likely to be successful than are therapies aimed at inhibiting the progression of the lesion at an earlier stage, or preferably even preventing the earliest lesion in the first place. To develop such strategies one must understand the natural history of the lesion and the pathogenetic events responsible for its development. Pathologists have long recognized several stages of human atherosclerosis, namely the fatty streak, the transitional lesion (also called the fibrofatty streak, the proliferative lesion or transitional lesion), and the plaque (6). Fatty streaks are found in the arterial beds of even young individuals in Western societies, and most investigators believe that these are the precursor of the transitional and more advanced lesion. If this is correct, then a detailed study of the pathogenesis of the fatty streak should give insights that might enable us to develop successful strategies to prevent its occurrence and or halt its progression to the transitional lesion.

Initial Steps in Lesion Formation

To study the initial steps in the formation of the fatty streak, one needs an animal model. As early as the late 19th century investigators observed that feeding cholesterol to laboratory animals, so that plasma levels were raised, caused formation of fatty streaks and even more complicated lesions. In recent years knowledge of this process has been advanced greatly by detailed studies of the morphological events that occur over time following initiation of cholesterol feeding in rabbits and nonhuman primates, as well as by similar studies in the genetically hypercholesterolemic WHHL rabbits (3,4,7–11). Although the "response to injury" hypothesis originally suggested that endothelial denudation was the earliest pathological event in the initiation of the fatty streak in response to cholesterol feeding, it is now recognized that such endothelial damage is not the initial event, but rather a subsequent event that contributes importantly to the development and progression of the fatty streak (7,8,12). In fact, in response to cholesterol feeding, the earliest event appears to be the focal accumulation of LDL within the subintimal space of an apparently "normal" artery (3,4). Within days of initiating dietary cholesterol, LDL begins to accumulate in selected sites within the arterial wall that are known to have a predilection for atherosclerosis (as opposed to sites that are relatively "resistant"). It should be emphasized that this subintimal focal accumulation of LDL occurs *prior* to any morphologic change in the overlying endothelium, and prior to the appearance of macrophages or smooth muscle cells in the intima. Furthermore, kinetic studies indicate that the "permeability" of the endothelium is not enhanced in these focal areas at this early stage, relative to lesion-resistant sites of the aorta, suggesting that localized factors within the extracellular matrix of these regions bind LDL and prevent its egress. This focal accumulation of LDL, at least in the cholesterol-fed rabbit, appears to be the first identifiable event in lesion-prone sites of the aorta (3,4).

Fatty Streak Formation

Shortly after this focal accumulation occurs, circulating monocytes begin to adhere to the luminal surface of the overlying endothelium (9,10). Monocytes are likely drawn to the focal areas of LDL accumulation by chemotactic factors, which may be direct or indirect consequences of oxidative modification of LDL, as noted below. In addition, the surface of the endothelium, which normally repels leukocytes, now contains surface ligands, which serve to specifically bind circulating monocytes (13). Subsequent to endothelial binding, monocytes, presumably drawn by chemoattractants, migrate into the subintimal space though gap junctions in adjacent endothelial cells. Again, it should be emphasized that at this early stage of lesion development, monocytes are still found within the subintimal space under an *intact* endothelium. Subsequently, they can be noted to begin to take the classic appearance of the "foam cell," which is due to enrichment of cholesteryl ester. Later, as more monocytes enter into these focal accumulations and more foam cells are generated, their volume increases and the endothelial cells overlying them may be stretched quite thin and actually rupture, exposing the underlying macrophages to the circulating blood elements (8). At this stage, platelets attach to monocytes as well as to the exposed structural components of the artery wall, and platelet aggregation and release can occur. Thus, the events envisioned in the original response-to-injury hypothesis can now take place with the release of factors such as PDGF, which serves both to recruit smooth muscles cells into the intimal layer and to stimulate their proliferation (12). At this point the events leading to initiation of the proliferative lesion have begun.

Lipid Accumulation in Macrophages

A key event in the sequence described above is conversion of circulating monocytes into arterial wall macrophages capable of ingesting large amounts of lipoproteins. Understanding the mechanisms by which this conversion takes place is crucial if one is to understand the origin of the fatty streak. Once monocytes become resident within the subintimal space their phenotypic expression is altered profoundly, yet little is known about the factors involved in this conversion; indeed, studies of this model of differentiation should yield fundamental insights into cell differentiation in general. Whatever these mechanisms are, once the monocyte has changed to a macrophage, it begins to rapidly take up LDL.

Several lines of evidence suggest that macrophage uptake of LDL does not occur to any significant extent by way of classic LDL-receptor pathways (14). First, exposure of macrophages to LDL in culture leads to downregulation of LDL receptors and thus, as in other cells, uptake of native LDL is downregulated. Second, in cell culture one cannot convert macrophages to foam cells simply by exposing them to native LDL. Third, humans with homozygous familial hypercholesterolemia (HFH), as well as the receptor-deficient WHHL rabbit—a model of HFH—develop severe and rapid atherosclerosis, with marked foam cell formation, despite a total lack of LDL receptors. If the LDL receptor is not involved in the uptake mechanism by which macrophages take up excessive amounts of LDL, what then accounts for foam cell formation? Resolution of this paradox was first suggested by Goldstein and co-workers (15) who noted that a primary function of macrophages is to remove denatured proteins. They showed that a chemical modification of LDL, acetylation, led to a negatively charged and modified LDL that now had a rapid uptake in cultured macrophage. This uptake mechanism was saturable, was not downregulated, and, in fact, could promote foam cell formation. This uptake was attributed to a distinct receptor, designated the "scavenger" or "acetyl-LDL receptor," found only on monocyte/macrophages, Kupffer cells, and some endothelial cells. This pathway also leads to the uptake of other chemically modified forms of LDL, such as the negatively charged malondialdehyde-conjugated LDL (16,17). At the time that these findings were made there was no evidence that such chemical modifications occurred to any extent *in vivo*. However, a biological modification that appears to be analogous to these chemical modifications has been described now.

THE ROLE OF MODIFIED LDL

In 1981 Henrikson and co-workers (18) found that when LDL was incubated with cultured endothelial cells for 18 hr it underwent striking physical and chemical changes, including the fact that such endothelial cell-modified LDL (EC-LDL) was taken up by cultured macrophages 2 to 4 times more rapidly than native LDL. Furthermore, native LDL did not compete for the uptake and degradation of EC-LDL, whereas acetyl LDL did. These data suggested that EC-LDL was being recognized, at least in part, by way of a scavenger receptor. More recent data suggest that a portion of the uptake and degradation of EC-LDL also occurs by way of yet another alternative high-affinity receptor (19). Subsequently, Henriksen et al. (20), as well as Heinecke et al. (21) and Morel et al. (22), showed that smooth muscle cells in culture also were able to effect a similar modification. In fact, more recent data have shown that monocyte-derived macrophages can themselves effect such modifications of LDL (23,24). Thus, *in vitro*, all three of the major cells types found in the artery wall can convert LDL to a modified form recognized by the scavenger receptor.

Attention then turned to defining the mechanism(s) by which LDL was altered to cause its recognition by the scavenger receptor. Steinbrecher et al. (25), Morel et al. (22), and Heinecke et al. (21) demonstrated that the cell-induced modification of LDL was initiated as the result of peroxidation of polyunsaturated fatty acids present in the LDL lipids, and that this was inhibited by the presence of antioxidants in the medium, such as butylated hydroxytoluene (BHT) or vitamin E. Furthermore, the oxidative modification was dependent on low concentrations of heavy metals in the medium, such as copper or iron, and could be inhibited completely by chelators such as EDTA. During oxidative modification, there is extensive conversion of lecithin to lysolecithin (lyso PC), apparently as the result of a phospholipase A_2 activity intrinsic to LDL that appears to prefer peroxidized fatty acids as substrate (26). Inhibitors of phospholipase A_2 block the generation of both lyso PC and lipid peroxides as well as subsequent biological modification. In addition, a large number of other as yet uncharacterized polar fatty acid products and sterols are generated that may have important biological consequences.

We now know that subsequent to the initiation of the peroxidation of fatty acids and activation of the phospholipase A_2 activity, there is the generation and release of a variety of fatty acid fragments, such as malondialdehyde (MDA) and 4-hydroxynonenal (4-HNE). These highly reactive fragments can form a complex with apo B, the protein of LDL, forming stable protein-lipid adducts. In addition, other changes occur in apo B, including cleavage into multiple fragments, presumably due to oxidative attack. As a result, neoepitopes are generated on LDL, the surface charge of the particle becomes more negative, and in some manner these changes lead to enhanced recognition by at least two different receptors on macrophages. This sequence of events is shown in Fig. 1.

In addition to having enhanced recognition and uptake by macrophages, leading to net cholesteryl ester deposition, oxidized LDL may contribute to atherogenesis by other mechanisms as well (Fig. 2). To a large extent, these other effects relate to the consequences of the variously oxidized fatty acid fragments and sterols formed during lipid peroxidation which are quite polar and can diffuse out of the LDL into adjacent cells or structures where they may exert important biological effects. For example, oxidized LDL is a potent chemotactic factor for monocytes and serves to attract monocytes into the subintimal

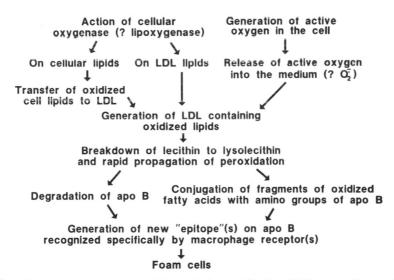

FIG. 1. Proposed mechanisms by which oxidative modification of LDL occurs. From ref. 2.

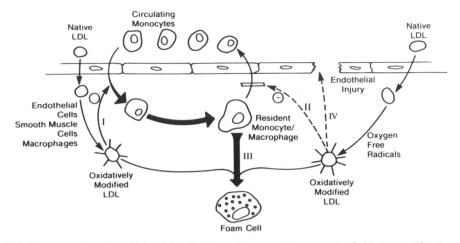

FIG. 2. Mechanisms by which oxidized LDL contribute to atherogenesis. Oxidative modification of LDL (catalyzed by endothelial cells, smooth muscle cells, or macrophages) presumably takes place in a protected environment of the subendothelial space. Products of oxidized LDL are chemotactic for monocytes (I) but inhibitory for macrophages (II). In addition, oxidized LDL is cytotoxic to endothelial cells and in subtoxic levels may affect gene expression (IV). Finally, oxidized LDL is taken up at an enhanced rate by macrophages, directly contributing to foam cell formation (III). From ref. 27.

space. Quinn et al. (27) have shown that lyso PC can account, in part, for this chemotactic activity. Furthermore, once monocytes have phenotypically changed to macrophages, oxidized LDL serves to inhibit their cellular movement, thus inhibiting their egress from the lesion. As a result, oxidized LDL serves to trap macrophages within the subintimal space. In addition, the cytotoxicity of oxidized LDL depends on the oxidation of LDL lipids (22,28–29). These lipid peroxidation products may cause cellular damage directly, as occurs with endothelial cells, as well as cause other cytotoxic or cytopathic effects indirectly in cells that are part of the subsequent events that lead to the more complex, advanced lesions. For example, these oxidation products may cause altered gene expression in affected cells by changing transcriptional or posttranscriptional events (30–31). Finally, such products may alter the hemodynamic properties of the artery wall, and recently it has been shown that oxidized LDL can alter the endothelial response to agonists that normally release endothelial-dependent relaxing factors (32). Thus, the presence of "oxidized LDL" in the artery wall could have profound consequences for the atherogenic process.

EVIDENCE FOR THE PRESENCE *IN VIVO* OF OXIDIZED LDL

The outline above suggests ways in which oxidized LDL could be atherogenic. However, this construct is based on a variety of *in vitro* studies, and it is important to demonstrate that oxidized LDL occurs *in vivo*. Recently, our group has shown that oxidized LDL can be demonstrated, in fact, in atherosclerotic arteries of rabbits and man (33–36). Several lines of evidence now have been developed to support this contention. First, LDL has been eluted gently from arterial sections taken from spontaneously hypercholesterolemic WHHL rabbits as well as from aortic sections obtained from human organ donors (34). From each aortic section, LDL was gently eluted and then characterized in depth. The LDL isolated from the atherosclerotic aortic sections (but not from the normal arteries) had many of the physical properties found in LDL oxidized *in vitro*. Thus, lesion LDL had increased electrophoretic mobility, contained more free cholesterol, had a higher percentage of lyso PC in the total phospholipids compared with control plasma LDL, and had extensive fragmentation of apo B, all properties typical of *in vitro* oxidized LDL.

A second line of evidence comes from the use of immunologic probes. A number of antisera and monoclonal antibodies specific for oxidation-specific epitopes present in oxidized LDL but absent in native LDL were prepared (33,35). These reagents were generated using models of oxidized LDL, i.e., MDA-conjugated LDL and 4-HNE-conjugated LDL. These are among the several modifications of apo B generated by oxidation of polyunsaturated fatty acids, which form a complex with ε-amino groups of lysine residues as noted above. The model-modified forms of LDL were injected into homologous species so that antibodies against native LDL were not generated. Thus, the antisera and monoclonal antibodies produced were specific to the lipid-protein adduct, i.e., MDA-lysine residues and 4-HNE-lysine residues. Western blot analysis of the isolated lesion LDL demonstrated that both the intact apo B-100 band and several of the apo B fragments generated during oxidative modification reacted strongly with these antisera, but LDL isolated from normal human intima or from plasma did not (33,34).

Third and most importantly, it was shown that LDL isolated from atherosclerotic aortic sections had enhanced uptake in macrophages and that this uptake was competed for by *in vitro* oxidized LDL, as well as by MDA-LDL and lesion LDL, but not by plasma LDL. Furthermore, lesion LDL, but not plasma LDL, could promote cholesteryl ester formation in cultured macrophages (34). Thus, lesion LDL greatly resembles *in vitro* oxidized LDL in its biological properties as well.

Fourth, when the immunological reagents were used to stain the intact artery wall, there was extensive localization of the oxidation-specific epitopes to atherosclerotic sections of the aorta but not normal aorta, confirming the *in vivo* presence of these oxidation products (33,36). Haberland et al. (37) and Boyd et al. (38) recently have also provided immunocytochemical evidence for the presence of oxidized LDL in the artery wall.

Fifth, we have shown previously that even minor modifications of autologous LDL render it highly immunogenic, and in fact used this strategy to generate the oxidation-specific antisera used in the studies above. Thus, the various neoepitopes generated during the process of oxidative modification of LDL, which obviously are present in the artery wall, should result in the generation of auto-antibodies to such modifications. Indeed, Palinski et al. (33) have shown the presence of such autoantibodies, at least to one such epitope of oxidized LDL, MDA-lysine adducts, in the serum of both rabbits and humans. In more recent studies, these human autoantibodies have been used to stain the sections of rabbit atherosclerotic aorta and showed very similar patterns of staining to that obtained with the induced MDA-lysine specific antisera prepared in rabbits and mice (36).

A sixth line of evidence supporting the *in vivo* presence of oxidized LDL comes from studies using the antioxidant compound probucol. Our laboratory showed several years ago that probucol was a potent antioxidant (39). Because it is highly lipophilic, it is carried in plasma in the core of lipoproteins, chiefly in LDL. Thus, it is strategically located to exert optimally an antioxidant effect for the lipids of LDL. We also showed that LDL isolated from human subjects on conventional doses of probucol was resistant to cell-induced modification of LDL when tested *in vitro* and even partially resistant to severe stress induced *in vitro* by incubation of LDL with copper ion alone (39). To test the ability of antioxidant therapy to inhibit the atherosclerotic process, Carew et al. (40) fed probucol to WHHL rabbits and showed that sufficient concentrations existed in their LDL to render it relatively resistant to oxidation as judged by *in vitro* oxidation assays. Probucol was fed to WHHL rabbits for 9 months and then the extent of their atherosclerosis was determined. This was compared to a control group as well as to a group of rabbits fed lovastatin to lower their cholesterol levels to a degree comparable to that achieved with probucol. The data showed conclusively that the probucol-treated animals had a marked reduction in their atherosclerosis that could not be explained by the degree of cholesterol lowering. Data from Kita et al. have confirmed these results (41). Furthermore, Carew et al. (40) clearly showed that uptake and degradation of LDL was specifically inhibited in atherosclerotic lesions but not in normal portions of the aorta, and that this was consistent with the view that macrophage uptake and degradation was inhibited specifically. Thus, evidence is now available that oxidized LDL is present in atherosclerotic tissue. Although its role in a quantitative sense remains to be determined, the intervention studies in rabbits suggest that it plays an important role in the atherogenic process.

In the discussion above we have focused on oxidative modification of LDL as one such postsecretory modification of LDL that may increase its atherogenicity. However, it is likely that a variety of such modifications occur that also render LDL more atherogenic. For example, during the process of oxidative modification, a variety of neoepitopes are generated that may lead to the generation of autoantibodies. If such immune complexes form in the artery wall, and, in turn, fix complement, then a cascade of immunological mechanisms may be initiated leading to enhanced uptake of such complexes by macrophages, in part mediated by way of Fc-receptor mechanisms. In addition, the activation of a variety of immune cells can lead to a classic inflammatory response with attendant tissue destruction, as discussed elsewhere in this volume. Similarly, other modifications of LDL trapped within the artery wall may occur also (2), including aggregation, formation of other kinds of complexes (e.g., as with matrix proteins) and modification by glucose as occurs with both short-term and long-term nonenzymatic glycation reactions (42). All of these processes, in turn, may alter the physical and chemical properties of LDL, changing its immunogenicity, and thereby enhancing its atherogenicity.

SUMMARY

A new paradigm has been proposed suggesting that a variety of modifications of LDL occur in the artery wall that enhance its atherogenicity. This hypothesis suggests that modified LDL is recognized as foreign by macrophages and therefore has enhanced uptake. One such modification, oxidative modification of LDL, appears to be particularly relevant, not only because it can lead to enhanced cholesteryl ester accumulation in macrophages due to a direct enhanced uptake of the particle, but also because its polar, oxidized lipids may diffuse out of the particle and profoundly affect localized cells and structures within the artery wall. In addition, by generation of neoepitopes, it may become immunogenic and elicit immune-mediated mechanisms, which may contribute further to the progression of the atherosclerotic lesion.

It is important for us to learn the details of these mechanisms because they offer the potential for therapeutic intervention. For example, if oxidation of LDL in the artery wall is quantitatively important, then inhibition of this process should be expected to retard the atherogenic process. Thus, new therapeutic strategies can be developed that could play an important adjunctive role in the treatment of atherosclerosis in addition to therapies designed to lower plasma cholesterol.

ACKNOWLEDGMENTS

This work was supported in part by Grant HL-14197 from the National Heart, Lung, and Blood Institute, NIH.

REFERENCES

1. Small DM. Progression and regression of atherosclerotic lesions. Insights from lipid physical biochemistry. *Arteriosclerosis* 1988;8:103–129.
2. Steinberg D, Parthasarathy S, Carew TE, Khoo JC, Witztum JL. Beyond cholesterol: Modifications of low density lipoprotein that increase its atherogenicity. *New Engl J Med* 1989;320:915–924.
3. Schwenke DC, Carew TE. Initiation of atherosclerotic lesions in cholesterol-fed rabbits. I. Focal increases in arterial LDL concentration precede development of fatty streak lesions. *Arteriosclerosis* 1989;9:895–907.

4. Schwenke DC, Carew TE. Initiation of atherosclerotic lesions in cholesterol-fed rabbits. II. Selective retention of LDL vs. selective increases in LDL permeability in susceptible sites of arteries. *Arteriosclerosis* 1989;9:908–918.
5. Witztum JL. Current approaches to drug therapy for the hypercholesterolemic patient. *Circulation* 1989;80:1101–1114.
6. Gown AM, Tsukada T, Ross R. Human atherosclerosis: immunocytochemical analysis of the cellular composition of human atherosclerotic lesions. *Am J Pathol* 1986;125:191–207.
7. Gerrity RG, Naito HK, Richardson M, Schwartz CJ. Dietary-induced atherogenesis in swine. *Am J Pathol* 1979;95:775–793.
8. Faggiotto A, Ross R, Harker L. Studies of hypercholesterolemia in the nonhuman primate. I. Changes that lead to fatty streak formation. *Arteriosclerosis* 1984;4:323–340.
9. Aqel NM, Ball RY, Waldman H, Mitchinson MJ. Monocytic origin of foam cells in human atherosclerotic plaques. *Atherosclerosis* 1984;53:265–271.
10. Rosenfeld ME, Tsukada T, Gown AM, Ross R. Fatty streak initiation in the WHHL and comparably hypercholesterolemic fat-fed rabbits. *Arteriosclerosis* 1987;1:9–23.
11. Wissler RW. Progression and regression of atherosclerotic lesions. *Adv Exp Med Biol* 1978;104: 77–109.
12. Ross R. The pathogenesis of atherosclerosis—an update. *New Engl J Med* 1986;314:418–500.
13. Bevilacqua MP, Pober JS, Wheeler ME, Cotran RS, Gimbrone MA Jr. Interleukin 1 acts on cultured human vascular endothelium to increase the adhesion of polymorphonuclear leukocytes, monocytes, and related leukocyte cell lines. *J Clin Invest* 1985;76:2003–2011.
14. Brown MS, Goldstein JL. Lipoprotein metabolism in the macrophage: implications for cholesterol deposition in atherosclerosis. *Ann Rev Biochem* 1983;52:223–261.
15. Goldstein JL, Ho YK, Basu SK, Brown MS. Binding site on macrophages that mediates uptake and degradation of acetylated low density lipoprotein, producing massive cholesterol deposition. *Proc Natl Acad Sci USA* 1979;76:333–337.
16. Fogelman AM, Schechter I, Seager J, Hokum M, Child JS, Edwards PE. Malondialdehyde alteration of low density lipoprotein leads to cholesterol accumulation in human monocyte-macrophages. *Proc Natl Acad Sci USA* 1980;74:2214–2218.
17. Haberland ME, Fogelman AM, Edwards PA. Specificity of receptor-mediated recognition of malondialdehyde-modified low density lipoproteins. *Proc Natl Acad Sci USA* 1982;79:1712–1716.
18. Henrikson T, Mahoney EM, Steinberg D. Enhanced macrophage degradation of low density lipoprotein previously incubated with cultured endothelial cells: recognition by the receptor for acetylated low density lipoproteins. *Proc Natl Acad Sci USA* 1981;78:6499–6503.
19. Sparrow CP, Parthasarathy S, Steinberg D. A macrophage receptor that recognizes oxidized LDL but not acetylated LDL. *J Biol Chem* 1989;264:2599–2604.
20. Henrikson T, Mahoney EM, Steinberg D. Enhanced macrophage degradation of biologically modified low density lipoprotein. *Arteriosclerosis* 1983;3:149–159.
21. Heinecke JW, Rosen H, Chait A. Iron and copper promote modification of low density lipoprotein by human arterial smooth muscle cells in culture. *J Clin Invest* 1984;74:1890–1894.
22. Morel DW, DiCorleto PE, Chisolm GM. Endothelial and smooth muscle cells alter low density lipoprotein *in vitro* by free radical oxidation. *Arteriosclerosis* 1984;4:357–364.
23. Cathcart MK, Morel DW, Chisolm GM. Monocytes and neutrophils oxidize low density lipoproteins making it cytotoxic. *J Leuk Biol* 1985;38:341–350.
24. Parthasarathy S, Printz DJ, Boyd D, Joy L, Steinberg D. Macrophage oxidation of low density lipoprotein generates a modified form recognized by the scavenger receptor. *Arteriosclerosis* 1986;6:505–510.
25. Steinbrecher UP, Parthasarathy S, Leake DS, Witztum JL, Steinberg D. Modification of low density lipoprotein by endothelial cells involves lipid peroxidation and degradation of low density lipoprotein phospholipids. *Proc Natl Acad Sci USA* 1984;83:3883–3887.
26. Parthasarathy S, Steinbrecher UP, Barnett J, Witztum JL, Steinberg D. Essential role of phospholipase A_2 activity in endothelial cell-induced modification of low density lipoprotein. *Proc Natl Acad Sci USA* 1985;82:3000–3004.
27. Quinn MT, Parthasarathy S, Fong LG, Steinberg D. Oxidatively modified low density lipoproteins: a potential role in recruitment and retention of monocyte/macrophages during atherogenesis. *Proc Natl Acad Sci USA* 1987;84:2995–2998.

28. Hessler JR, Robertson AL Jr, Chisolm GM. LDL-induced cytotoxicity and its inhibition by HDL in human vascular smooth muscle and endothelial cells in culture. *Atherosclerosis* 1979;32:213–229.
29. Henriksen T, Evensen SA, Paulander B. Injury to human endothelial cells in culture induced by low density lipoproteins. *Scand J Clin Lab Invest* 1979;39:361–368.
30. Rajavashisth TB, Berliner JA, Andalabi A, et al. Minimally modified LDL induces the expression of M-CSF, GM-CSF, and G-CSF by Cultured Aortic Endothelial Cells. *Circulation* 1989;80 II:163.
31. Fox PL, Chisolm GM, DiCorleto PE. Lipoprotein-mediated inhibition of endothelial cell production of platelet-derived growth factor-like protein depends on free radical lipid peroxidation. *J Biol Chem* 1987;262:6046–6054.
32. Kugiyama K, Bucay M, Morrisett JD, Roberts R, Henry PD. Oxidized LDL impairs endothelium-dependent arterial relaxation. *Circulation* 1989;80 II:279.
33. Palinski W, Rosenfeld ME, Ylä-Herttuala S, et al. Low density lipoprotein undergoes oxidative modification in vivo. *Proc Natl Acad Sci USA* 1989;86:1372–1376.
34. Ylä-Herttuala S, Palinski W, Rosenfeld ME, et al. Evidence for the presence of oxidatively modified low density lipoprotein in atherosclerotic lesions of rabbit and man. *J Clin Invest* 1980;84:1086–1095.
35. Palinski W, Ylä-Herttuala S, Rosenfeld ME, et al. Antisera and monoclonal antibodies specific for epitopes generated during the oxidative modification of low density lipoproteins. *Arteriosclerosis* 1990; May–June.
36. Rosenfeld ME, Palinski W, Ylä-Herttuala S, Butler SW, Witztum JL. Distribution of oxidized proteins and apolipoprotein B in atherosclerotic lesions of varying severity from WHHL rabbits: immunocytochemical analysis using antibodies generated against modified and native LDL. *Arteriosclerosis* 1990; May–June.
37. Haberland ME, Fong D, Cheng L. Malondialdehyde-altered protein occurs in atheroma of Watanabe heritable hyperlipidemic rabbits. *Science* 1988;241:215–218.
38. Boyd HC, Gown AM, Wolfbayer G, Chait A. Direct evidence for a protein recognized by a monoclonal antibody against oxidatively modified LDL in atherosclerotic lesions from Watanabe Heritable Hyperlipemic rabbit. *Am J Pathol* 1988;135:1372–1376.
39. Parthasarathy S, Young SG, Witztum JL, Pittman RC, Steinberg D. Probucol inhibits oxidative modification of low density lipoprotein. *J Clin Invest* 1986;77:641–644.
40. Carew TE, Schwenke DC, Steinberg D. Antiatherogenic effect of probucol unrelated to its hypocholesterolemic effect: evidence that antioxidants *in vivo* can selectively inhibit low density lipoprotein degradation in macrophage-rich fatty streaks slowing the progression of atherosclerosis in the WHHL rabbit. *Proc Natl Acad Sci USA* 1987;84:7725–7729.
41. Kita T, Nagano Y, Yokode M, et al. Probucol prevents the progression of atherosclerosis in Watanabe heritable hyperlipidemic rabbit, an animal model for familial hypercholesterolemia. *Proc Natl Acad Sci USA* 1987;84:5928–5931.
42. Witztum JL, Koschinsky T. Metabolic and immunological consequences of glycation of low density lipoproteins. In: Baynes JW, Monnier VM, eds. *The Maillard reaction in aging, diabetes, and nutrition.* New York: Alan R. Liss, Inc. 1989:219–234.

Atherosclerosis Reviews, Volume 21,
edited by A. Leaf and P. C. Weber.
Raven Press, Ltd., New York © 1990.

Platelet–Vessel Wall Interactions:

Eicosanoids and EDRF

Salvador Moncada, Richard M. J. Palmer, and E. Annie Higgs

*The Wellcome Research Laboratories, Langley Court,
Beckenham, Kent BR3 3BS, England*

The importance of the vascular endothelium in vessel wall homeostasis has become apparent in recent years with the discovery of prostacyclin and endothelium-derived relaxing factor (EDRF). Both of these are produced by vascular endothelium and are potent vasodilators and inhibitors of platelet aggregation. The more we understand of the actions and interactions of these two substances and of their role as regulators of vascular tone and platelet–vessel wall interactions, the greater is our knowledge of the physiology and pathophysiology of the cardiovascular system.

VASCULAR PRODUCTION OF PROSTACYCLIN

Prostacyclin is a metabolite of arachidonic acid that is released from the vessel wall in response to mechanical, immunological, or chemical stimuli as well as trauma. Although smooth muscle cells can also convert arachidonic acid to prostacyclin, the endothelial cells are its chief source in the vessel wall.

Prostacyclin is a vasodilator and the most potent naturally occurring inhibitor of platelet aggregation yet discovered. It is chemically unstable, with a half-life of 2 to 3 min, breaking down to 6-keto-PGF$_{1\alpha}$ (1). The inhibition of platelet aggregation by prostacyclin is correlated with an activation of the adenylate cyclase system, leading to a substantial rise in platelet intracellular cyclic AMP levels. Other properties of prostacyclin include cytoprotection, enhanced fibrinolysis, and stimulation of cholesterol metabolism (2).

A number of diseases, such as atherosclerosis, have been associated with impaired prostacyclin production. Reduced prostacyclin formation by atherosclerotic vascular tissue has been demonstrated both in experimental animals and in humans. Aortas from rabbits made atherosclerotic by cholesterol feeding show a transient increase followed by a reduction in prostacyclin production (3).

Atherosclerosis, however, is not associated invariably with reduced generation of prostacyclin as there have been reports of increased release of prostacyclin or a metabolite, both in experimental models of atherosclerosis (4) and in patients with severe diffuse atherosclerosis (5). This may be the result of the release from activated platelets of factors, such as 5-hydroxytryptamine and platelet-activating factor, with potential prostacyclin-releasing properties. Thus, it is possible that an overall decrease in the ability to release prostacyclin by vascular endothelial cells may coexist with an increased production due to pathological stimulation.

Prostacyclin has been shown to have a regulatory role in aortic cholesterol metabolism. In cultured vascular smooth muscle cells prostacyclin at low concentrations increases the activity of the enzymes that metabolize cholesteryl esters (6). In human atherosclerotic smooth muscle cells in culture, cholesteryl ester metabolism is enhanced by two stable prostacyclin analogs so that the triglyceride and cholesteryl ester levels in the cells are reduced substantially (7).

Prostacyclin also can inhibit mobilization of fibrinogen-binding sites on human platelets *in vitro,* which thus may limit the extent of fibrinogen-platelet interactions. In addition, prostacyclin enhances fibrinolytic activity in several tissues by inducing the protease plasminogen activator, a process which could contribute to its long-term clinical actions in chronic obstructive diseases of the circulation (8).

Prostacyclin has been shown to inhibit the release of mitogenic activity ("growth factors") from stimulated human platelets (9). Such growth factors are thought to mediate the progression of atherosclerosis by promoting smooth muscle cell and fibroblast proliferation (10).

The use of prostacyclin, as a stable freeze-dried preparation, has been studied in many clinical conditions (11,12). In addition to its use in extracorporeal circulation systems such as cardiopulmonary bypass operations, renal dialysis, and charcoal hemoperfusion, prostacyclin has been shown to be effective in the treatment of atherosclerotic peripheral vascular disease and Raynaud's syndrome. Also, it has been tested in the treatment of other thrombotic conditions such as stroke and myocardial infarction. Prostacyclin has been used in patients with pulmonary hypertension and has been found to have pulmonary hemodynamic effects similar to those of hydralazine and nifedipine. What is becoming clear is that the efficacy of prostacyclin, particularly its long-lasting effect in certain clinical conditions such as peripheral vascular disease and Raynaud's syndrome, cannot be explained solely in terms of its short-lasting vasodilator and antiaggregatory actions. Consequently, interest is being focused on the other activities of prostacyclin such as cytoprotection, fibrinolysis, and stimulation of cholesterol metabolism.

IDENTIFICATION OF A NEW BIOCHEMICAL PATHWAY

In 1980 Furchgott and Zawadzki demonstrated the existence of a humoral factor, later known as endothelium-derived relaxing factor (EDRF), which mediates endothelium-dependent relaxation in vascular tissue (13). This newly recognized labile mediator was shown by bioassay studies to be inactivated by superoxide anions and to be protected from breakdown by superoxide dismutase. In addition to its vasodilator properties, EDRF was found to inhibit platelet aggregation, to induce disaggregation of aggregated platelets, and to inhibit platelet adhesion. All these properties are mediated by activation of the soluble guanylate cyclase, leading to elevated cyclic GMP levels within the smooth muscle cell or the platelet (14–16).

Following the suggestion in 1986 by Furchgott (17) and Ignarro (18) that EDRF may be nitric oxide (NO) or a closely related species, we compared the pharmacological properties of EDRF and NO on vascular smooth muscle and on platelets and found them to be identical (19). Furthermore, using a chemiluminescence method for measuring NO, we have demonstrated that vascular endothelial cells in culture release sufficient NO to account for the effects of EDRF on vascular strips, platelet aggregation, and adhesion (19,20). These findings have been confirmed subsequently using other methods of chemical detection of NO. These biological and chemical data, considered together, demonstrate that EDRF is NO.

We went on to show that vascular endothelial cells synthesize NO from the terminal guanido nitrogen atom(s) of L-arginine (21). This reaction is specific as several analogs of L-arginine are not substrates and are inhibited in a dose-dependent and enantiomerically specific manner by N^G-monomethyl-L-arginine (L-NMMA) (21,22).

BIOLOGICAL IMPORTANCE OF NITRIC OXIDE

The identification and characterization of L-NMMA as a specific inhibitor of the endothelial NO synthase has allowed the importance of the formation of NO from L-arginine to be studied *in vitro*. L-NMMA inhibits the stimulated release of NO from endothelial cells in culture (23) and from perfused vascular tissue (22,23). It also causes an endothelium-dependent increase in the tone of vascular tissue (23) and inhibits endothelium-dependent relaxation induced by various agents (22–24). Furthermore, in the isolated perfused rabbit heart, L-NMMA causes a rise in coronary perfusion pressure and an inhibition of the vasodilatation induced by acetycholine (ACh). This is accompanied by inhibition of the release of NO into the coronary effluent (25).

Studies on the effect of L-NMMA on the blood pressure of anesthetized rabbits revealed that intravenous administration of L-NMMA, but not N^G-monomethyl-D-arginine (D-NMMA), induced an increase in blood pressure, which was associated with a reduced release *ex vivo* of NO from the perfused aorta of treated animals (26). Furthermore, the fall in blood pressure induced by ACh was also inhibited by L-NMMA. All these effects were enantiomerically specific and were reversed or abolished by L-arginine. Subsequently, L-NMMA has been shown to cause a rise in blood pressure in anesthetized guinea pigs (27) and rats (28). These results show that the vasculature is constantly utilizing L-arginine for the generation of NO, which plays a role in the maintenance of blood pressure.

The effects of L-NMMA on regional blood flow have been studied in conscious, chronically instrumented rats (29). Vascular conductance was reduced to a similar extent (up to 60%) in the renal, mesenteric, internal carotid, and hindquarters by L-NMMA, indicating the critical role of NO formation from L-arginine in the maintenance of regional blood flow.

Studies using L-NMMA in the brachial artery (30) and in the veins of the dorsal part of the hand (31) of humans revealed that there is a basal formation of NO from L-arginine which contributes to the resting tone in the arterial circulation, but not in the venous circulation. This indicates differences in the importance of the L-arginine:NO pathway in regulating tone in different parts of the circulation. In both the arterial and the venous circulation, however, mediator-induced vasodilatation was dependent on the formation of NO from L-arginine (30,31).

Nitric oxide, like prostacyclin, is a potent inhibitor of platelet activation *in vitro* (16,20). Prostacyclin and NO potentiate each other's actions as inhibitors of platelet aggregation and inducers of platelet disaggregation. The inhibitory actions of prostacyclin and NO can be differentiated clearly, however, because those of prostacyclin are mediated via cyclic AMP, whereas those of NO are mediated via cyclic GMP. It is possible that the low concentrations of prostacyclin found in plasma may have a physiological effect in regulating platelet aggregability if acting on a background of NO release. The physiological significance of the antiaggregatory actions of NO remains to be investigated, although there are reports that endogenous NO inhibits platelet function *in vivo* (32,33).

Nitric oxide, unlike prostacyclin, is a potent inhibitor of platelet adhesion via an effect on cyclic GMP (34). Because the small effect of prostacyclin on adhesion is related to an effect on cyclic GMP, it may be that cyclic GMP levels regulate membrane properties responsible for cell adhesion, in general (34). The fact that there is no synergistic interaction between NO and prostacyclin on platelet adhesion also suggests that the physiological process of platelet adhesion and repair of the vessel wall may proceed in circumstances in which both substances are interacting to exert a powerful antithrombotic action.

PATHOLOGICAL IMPLICATIONS OF NITRIC OXIDE

The ability of the endothelium to constantly generate NO, which controls vessel wall diameter and consequently plays a decisive role as a determinant of blood flow and blood pressure, adds an important mechanism to be considered when analyzing phenomena such as hyperemia, autoregulation, flow-dependent dilatation, blood pressure regulation, and mechanisms for edema formation in the cardiovascular system. Indeed, NO can be considered the endogenous nitrovasodilator, the actions of which are imitated by compounds such as nitroglycerin that have been in clinical use for over 100 years (35). This discovery will give new impetus to the search for compounds which either imitate its actions or increase its production in the cardiovascular system.

A diminished vasodilator response to ACh has been reported in animal models of hypertension (35), hyperlipidemia (35), diabetes (36), human atherosclerosis, and coronary artery disease (37,38). Decreased production of NO by the endothelium could account for these observations. Furthermore, reduced NO production could lead to the enhanced adhesion of platelets to the vessel wall observed in these conditions, and lack of NO may also be involved in the development of vasospasm and restenosis after angioplasty. It is not yet known whether NO in the vessel wall modulates white cell activation, regulates enzymes involved in cholesterol metabolism as does prostacyclin, or controls smooth muscle proliferation. Nitric oxide, like prostacyclin is cytoprotective (39). It remains to be established whether, as in aggregation, NO and prostacyclin act synergistically as cytoprotectors. Further studies on the effects and the interactions between NO and prostacyclin will, without doubt, help to clarify the thromboresistant properties of vascular endothelium as well as its changes during pathological phenomena.

REFERENCES

1. Moncada S. Biological importance of prostacyclin. *Br J Pharmacol* 1982;76:3–31.
2. Moncada S. Prostacyclin—Discovery and biological importance. In: Longenecker GL, Schaffer SW, eds. *Prostaglandins: research and clinical update.* Minneapolis: Alpha Editions, 1985;1–39.
3. Beetens JR, Coene M-C, Verheyen A, Zonnekeyn L, Herman AG. Biphasic response of intimal prostacyclin production during the development of experimental atherosclerosis. *Prostaglandins* 1986;32:319–334.
4. Tremoli E, Socini A, Petroni A, Galli C. Increased platelet aggregability is associated with increased prostacyclin production by vessel walls in hypercholesterolemic rabbits. *Prostaglandins* 1982;24:397–404.
5. Fitzgerald GA, Smith B, Pedersen AK, Brash, AR. Increased prostacyclin biosynthesis in patients with severe atherosclerosis and platelet activation. *N Engl J Med* 1984;310:1065–1068.
6. Hajjar DP, Weksler BB. Metabolic activity of cholesteryl esters in aortic smooth muscle cells is altered by prostaglandins I_2 and E_2. *J Lipid Res* 1983;24:1176–1185.
7. Orekhov AN, Tertov VV, Masurov AV, Andreeva ER, Repin VS, Smirnov VN. "Regression" of atherosclerosis in cell culture: effects of stable prostacyclin analogues. *Drug Dev Res* 1986;9:189–201.
8. Moncada S, Higgs EA. Arachidonate metabolism in blood cells and the vessel wall. *Clin Haematol* 1986;15:273–292.
9. Willis AL, Smith DL, Vigo C, Kluge AF. Effects of prostacyclin and orally active stable mimetic agent RS-93427-007 on basic mechanisms of atherogenesis. *Lancet* 1986;2:682–683.
10. Ross R. The pathogenesis of atherosclerosis—an update. *N Engl J Med* 1986;314:488–500.
11. Moncada S, Higgs EA. Prostaglandins in the pathogenesis and prevention of vascular disease. *Blood Rev* 1987;1:141–145.
12. Moncada S. Clinical use of prostacyclin. In: Triger DR, ed. *Advanced medicine vol. 22.* London: Baillere Tindall. 1986:323–332.

13. Furchgott RF, Zawadzki JV. The obligatory role of endothelial cells in the relaxation of arterial smooth muscle by acetylcholine. *Nature* 1980;288:373–376.
14. Furchgott RF. The role of endothelium in the responses of vascular smooth muscle to drugs. *Ann Rev Pharmacol Toxicol* 1984;24:175–197.
15. Griffith TM, Edwards DH, Lewis MJ, Newby AC, Henderson AH. The nature of endothelium-derived vascular relaxant factor. *Nature* 1984;308:645–647.
16. Moncada S, Palmer RMJ, Higgs EA. Prostacyclin and endothelium-derived relaxing factor: biological interactions and significance. In: Verstraete M, Vermylen J, Lijnen HR, Arnout J, eds. *Thrombosis and haemostasis.* Leuven, Belgium: Leuven University Press, 1987:587–618.
17. Furchgott RF. Studies on relaxation of rabbit aorta by sodium nitrite: the basis for the proposal that the acid-activatable inhibitory factor from retractor penis is inorganic nitrite and the endothelium-derived relaxing factor is nitric oxide. In: Vanhoutte PM, ed. *Vasodilatation: vascular smooth muscle, peptides, autonomic nerves and endothelium.* New York: Raven Press, 1988: 401–414.
18. Ignarro LJ, Byrns RE, Wood KS. Biochemical and pharmacological properties of endothelium-derived relaxing factor and its similarity to nitric oxide radicals. In: Vanhoutte PM, ed. *Vasodilatation: vascular smooth muscle, peptides, autonomic nerves and endothelium.* New York: Raven Press, 1988:427–436.
19. Palmer RMJ, Ferrige AG, Moncada S. Nitric oxide release accounts for the biological activity of endothelium-derived relaxing factor. *Nature* 1987;327:524–526.
20. Moncada S, Radomski MW, Palmer, RMJ. Endothelium-derived relaxing factor: identification as nitric oxide and role in the control of vascular tone and platelet function. *Biochem Pharmacol* 1988;37:2495–2501.
21. Palmer, RMJ, Ashton DS, Moncada S. Vascular endothelial cells synthesize nitric oxide from L-arginine. *Nature* 1988;333:664–666.
22. Palmer RMJ, Rees DD, Ashton DS, Moncada S. L-arginine is the physiological precursor for the formation of nitric oxide in endothelium-dependent relaxation. *Biochem Biophys Res Commun* 1988;153:1251–1256.
23. Rees DD, Palmer RMJ, Hodson HF, Moncada S. A specific inhibitor of nitric oxide formation from L-arginine attenuates endothelium-dependent relaxation. *Br J Pharmacol* 1989;96:418–424.
24. Sakuma I, Stuehr DJ, Gross SS, Nathan C, Levi R. Identification of arginine as a precursor of endothelium-derived relaxing factor (EDRF). *Proc Natl Acad Sci USA* 1988;85:8664–8667.
25. Amezcua J-L, de Souza BM, Palmer RMJ, Moncada S. Inhibition of nitric oxide synthesis inhibits endothelium-dependent vasodilatation in the rabbit isolated heart. *Br J Pharmacol* 1989;97:1119–1124.
26. Rees DD, Palmer RMJ, Moncada S. Role of endothelium-derived nitric oxide in the regulation of blood pressure. *Proc Natl Acad Sci USA* 1989;86:3375–3378.
27. Aisaka K, Gross SS, Griffith OW, Levi R. N^G-methylarginine, an inhibitor of endothelium-derived nitric oxide synthesis, is a potent pressor agent in the guinea pig: does nitric oxide regulate blood pressure in vivo? *Biochem Biophys Res Commun* 1989;160:881–886.
28. Whittle BJR, Lopez-Belmonte J, Rees DD. Modulation of the vasodepressor actions of acetylcholine, bradykinin, substance P and endothelium in the rat by a specific inhibitor of nitric oxide formation. *Br J Pharmacol* 1989;98:646–652.
29. Gardiner SM, Compton AM, Bennett T, Palmer RMJ, Moncada S. Control of regional blood flow by endothelium-derived nitric oxide. *Hypertension* 1990; 15 (in press).
30. Vallance P, Collier J, Moncada S. Effects of endothelium-derived nitric oxide on peripheral arteriolar tone in man. *Lancet* 1989;2:997–1000.
31. Vallance P, Collier J, Moncada S. Nitric oxide synthesised from L-arginine mediates endothelium-dependent dilatation in human veins in vivo. *Cardiovasc Res* 1989;23:1053–1057.
32. Hogan JC, Lewis MJ, Henderson AH. *In vivo* EDRF activity influences platelet function. *Br J Pharmacol* 1988;94:1020–1022.
33. Bhardwaj R, Page CP, May GR, Moore PK. Endothelium-derived relaxing factor inhibits platelet aggregation in human whole blood in vitro and in the rat in vivo. *Eur J Pharmacol* 1988;157: 83–91.
34. Radomski MW, Palmer RMJ, Moncada S. The role of nitric oxide and cGMP in platelet adhesion to vascular endothelium. *Biochem Biophys Res Commun* 1987;148:1482–1489.

35. Moncada S, Palmer RMJ, Higgs EA. The discovery of nitric oxide as the endogenous nitrovasodilator. *Hypertension* 1988;12:365–372.
36. Durante W, Sen AK, Sunahara FA. Impairment of endothelium-dependent relaxation in aortae from spontaneously diabetic rats. *Br J Pharmacol* 1988;94:463–468.
37. Ludmer PL, Selwyn AP, Shook TL, et al. Paradoxical vasoconstriction induced by acetylcholine in atherosclerotic coronary arteries. *N Engl J Med* 1986;315:1046–1051.
38. Bossaller C, Habib GB, Yamamoto H, Williams C, Wells S, Henry PD. Impaired muscarinic endothelium-dependent relaxation and cyclic guanosine 5'-monophosphate formation in atherosclerotic human coronary artery and rabbit aorta. *J Clin Invest* 1987;79:170–174.
39. Radomski MW, Palmer RMJ, Read NG, Moncada S. Isolation and washing of human platelets with nitric oxide. *Thromb Res* 1988;50:537–546.

Atherosclerosis Reviews, Volume 21,
edited by A. Leaf and P. C. Weber.
Raven Press, Ltd., New York © 1990.

Inflammatory and Immune Mechanisms in Atherogenesis

Peter Libby

*Departments of Medicine (Cardiology) and Cellular and Molecular Physiology and the
USDA Human Nutrition Research Center on Aging, Tufts University, and
New England Medical Center, Boston, Massachusetts 02111*

Current knowledge has challenged the classical view of atheroma as mere inanimate collections of insudated lipids. The results of modern studies emphasize the dynamic nature of these lesions produced by complex interactions between cells and chemical mediators, and have renewed interest in inflammatory and immune processes in atherogenesis (1–2). For example, application of monoclonal antibody technology has confirmed the long suspected presence of mononuclear phagocytes in atheroma (4–7). More surprisingly, this approach has disclosed prominent T-lymphocyte infiltration in complicated human athcroma (6–8). Other studies have established that blood vessel wall cells can both elaborate and respond to potent mediators of inflammatory and immune responses heretofore believed to exchange signals exclusively among leukocytes (9,10). A number of these mediators can modulate proliferation of smooth muscle cells, findings that relate these more recent findings to earlier searches for factors that control the growth of these cells (11–13). The interaction of lipoproteins with mononuclear phagocytes has received much attention (14,15). However, carnest pursuit of links between lipid metabolism and inflammatory and immune responses is just beginning. This review aims to illustrate the general points raised above with results from a number of laboratories. We will attempt to provide a synthesis that will highlight what is known as well as major outstanding and unresolved points in relation to the involvement of inflammatory and immune responses in atherogenesis.

INFLAMMATORY RESPONSES IN THE INITIATION OF ATHEROSCLEROSIS

Delineation of the initial events in human atherogenesis presents obvious difficulties. A number of important efforts under way are aimed at studying arterial lesions in juveniles who come to autopsy for various reasons. These studies have disclosed mononuclear phagocytes within the arterial wall even in young individuals (16,17). It remains uncertain whether the "fatty streak," a macrophage-rich lesion found in the arteries of children, represents the precursor to the complicated atheromatous plaque (18).

In light of the evident difficulties in studying the early events in formation of human atheromata, production of arterial lesions in animals has proven useful. Various strategies including dietary modification and mechanical manipulation such as balloon inflation can induce arterial pathology (19). The responses to and susceptibility of particular species to these interventions vary considerably. In every case the experimentally produced arterial lesions differ substantially from spontaneous human atheroma. A common approach to lesion induction, consumption of diets enriched in cholesterol and saturated fat, yields hyperlipoproteinemic states both quantitatively and qualitatively quite distinct from those encountered in most human patients with atherosclerosis. Despite all of these reservations, certain points emerge with sufficient consistency from studies performed on diverse species with various methods to command attention. In response to atherogenic diets, mononuclear phagocytes adhere to the intimal surface. These leukocytes then appear to diapedese into the intima and take up residence within the arterial wall where they accumulate lipid, a sequence common to hypercholesterolemic rabbits, swine, rats, and monkeys (20–23).

The reasons that monocytes adhere selectively to predictable foci on the luminal surface of the intima remain obscure. In many hyperlipidemic animal preparations, early accumulations of lipid-laden macrophages (resembling human fatty streaks) localize at flow dividers and other areas in which hydrodynamics may be altered. The precise hydrodynamic conditions that predispose to formation of such lesions remain controversial. There is disagreement on whether shear stress is increased or decreased at such sites. The wall tension or stretch in such focal areas also may help to determine susceptibility to fatty streak formation (24). Not only is there uncertainty regarding the hydrodynamic differences between lesional areas and unaffected regions, but little is known of mechanical-biochemical coupling. Endothelial cells contain stretch-activated ion channels that are likely candidates for transducing hydrodynamic alterations into changes in cell behavior (25–27). Such findings provide the basis for future physiologic–biochemical experiments that should clarify these issues.

Tissue culture studies have enabled major advances in understanding the mechanism of leukocyte association with endothelial cells. Under usual circumstances in vitro, endothelial cells exhibit relatively low adhesion for leukocytes. However, exposure of endothelial cells to certain well-defined inflammatory mediators increases their ability to bind leukocytes of various classes. (28,29). Treatment of leukocytes with some of the same stimuli also can influence their adhesivity for endothelium (30,31). These findings led to the postulate that endothelial cells could express on their surface, in an inducible fashion, specific leukocyte adhesion molecules that govern their interaction with these cells.

Recent studies of one such molecule, endothelial leukocyte adhesion molecule-1 (ELAM-1) illustrate this paradigm. This molecule appears to function as a specific receptor for polymorphonuclear leukocytes (32). In contrast to many intracellular adhesion molecules, the expression of this gene appears restricted to endothelial cells *in vivo.* Its structure has defined a new family of intracellular adhesion molecules distinct from the immunoglobulin superfamily-related cellular adhesion molecules (NCAMs and ICAMs). ELAM-1 is a transmembrane glycoprotein with regional sequence resemblances to certain lectins and complement regulatory proteins. Another recently defined molecule denoted GMP-140 or PADGEM, originally found on platelets, also occurs on endothelium and can bind leukocytes (33,34). Other members of the endothelial–leukocyte adhesion molecule functional family will soon emerge. In light of the consistent early increased adhesion of mononuclear cells to endothelial cells in response to atherogenic diets, the regulation of a putative monocyte-specific ELAM should prove particularly illuminating.

INFLAMMATORY MECHANISMS AND EVOLUTION OF THE NASCENT ATHEROSCLEROTIC LESION TO THE COMPLICATED PLAQUE

After adherence to the endothelium, experimental studies suggest that these cells migrate into a subendothelial location. The factors that govern this directed migration are characterized incompletely. Activities extractable from atherosclerotic lesions can stimulate monocyte chemokinesis (35–37). One such activity (human monocyte chemoattractant protein-1, MCP-1), expressed by various cell types including vascular wall cells, shares sequence similarity to the well-known platelet-derived growth factor (PDGF)–inducible gene JE (37–39). PDGF and other mediators implicated in atherogenesis may provide a chemotactic stimulus to cell locomotion into the intima also.

The association between hyperlipoproteinemia and monocyte-derived foam cell formation is advancing. The major form of lipoprotein circulating in response to most atherogenic diets is beta very-low-density lipoprotein (β-VLDL). Early arterial lesions in the Watanabe rabbit (a mutant strain whose serum LDL increases due to a deficiency in LDL receptors) also accumulate monocytes, as do rabbits fed an atherogenic diet that produces comparable levels of hypercholesterolemia (40,41). Indeed, both β-VLDL and LDL appear to share a common receptor on most cells (42). However, mononuclear cells express this receptor (the "apo BE" receptor) in relatively low levels, and exposure to ligands efficiently suppresses the expression of this receptor (14). A lower affinity but high capacity and constitutively expressed receptor for "modified" lipoproteins denoted the "scavenger" receptor probably accounts for entry of lipoproteins into monocytes during foam cell formation (43). The ligands used to characterize this receptor include LDL conjugated with acetyl groups or other moieties such as malondialdehyde. Oxidatively modified lipoproteins constitute potential endogenous ligands for this receptor. Exposure of LDL to various cell types and conditions that may be encountered *in vivo* in the arterial wall can lead to modifications that render LDL an appropriate substrate for the "scavenger" receptor (15).

So far we have reviewed how leukocytes may adhere, enter, and accumulate lipid within the nascent atheroma. A major outstanding question regarding lesion evolution concerns the degree of activation of these lipid-laden macrophages that have taken up residence within the arterial wall. This point is important, as expression of activated functions by these phagocytes could explain the eventual progression of fatty lesions to complicated fibrocalcific atheromata. For example, activated mononuclear phagocytes can elaborate a number of mediators that stimulate smooth muscle cell proliferation and may hasten fibrogenesis. These messengers include PDGF, transforming growth factor-α, and interleukin-1 (11,12,44–46). Another outstanding issue in regard to lesion formation is the relevance of the sequence of events well described in experimental animals to the formation of "spontaneous" human atherosclerosis. As emphasized above, we have only glimpses of the morphology of the earliest stages of human atherosclerosis. Perhaps a fusion of experimental results and modern advances in microanalysis of gene expression will permit testing of focused hypotheses in human lesions in the future to explore the relevance of the animal data to humans.

EVIDENCE FOR IMMUNOLOGICAL ACTIVITY IN THE ESTABLISHED HUMAN ATHEROSCLEROTIC LESION

Classical immunohistopathologic analysis of human atheromata suggested that accumulation of smooth muscle cells and mononuclear phagocytes characterized these lesions. The advent of monoclonal antibody technology placed the identification of cell types within complicated human atheromata on a firmer basis. Use of this technology has confirmed the presence of smooth muscle cells and macrophages. As noted above, one surprising finding was the previously unsuspected infiltration of T-lymphocytes particularly in the "shoulder" regions of mature human atheroma (6–8).

Another unexpected finding was the presence of smooth muscle cells bearing class II histocompatibility antigens (47,48). Until fairly recently, the ability to express this type of transplantation antigen was thought to be limited to bone marrow-derived leukocytes. Recognition of nominal antigens by helper T-cells during the initiation of the cellular immune response requires surface expression of class II histocompatibility antigens (HLA-DR, DP, and DQ). It is now known that a variety of nonleukocytic cells also may express class II antigens in some circumstances (49–51). The best established inducer of human class II antigen expression is the lymphokine γ-interferon (IFN-γ), a product of activated T-lymphocytes. The finding of T-cells in the atheroma adjacent to smooth muscle cells bearing class II antigens implied that some of the T-lymphocytes must be activated to secrete IFN-γ. Indeed, Hansson and colleagues have demonstrated recently that T-cells within the atherosclerotic lesions express IL-2 receptors, a direct indication of their state of activation (52). Furthermore, this laboratory demonstrated the presence of IFN-γ within human atheroma by immunohistochemical staining (52). The stimuli that activate T-lymphocytes remain a major unresolved issue in understanding the inflammatory nature in human atheromata. In addition to inducing macrophage functions and class II gene expression, IFN-γ can inhibit smooth muscle cell proliferation induced by serum, PDGF, or IL1. Thus, local evolution of IFN-γ may provide another link between inflammation, the immune response, and atherogenesis.

INFLAMMATORY MEDIATORS AND THE TRANSITION FROM CHRONIC TO ACUTE PHASES OF ATHEROSCLEROTIC DISEASE

Human atherosclerotic plaques commonly evolve for many years without provoking symptoms. The clinical manifestations due to interference with blood supply generally do not occur until mid to late life, although lesion formation usually begins much earlier. In many cases of atherosclerosis, the initial manifestations include transient symptoms such as angina pectoris, transient cerebral ischemic attacks, and intermittent claudication of the extremities. These episodic attacks often presage the dreaded life-threatening complications of atherosclerotic disease of the various circulations (e.g., acute myocardial infarction, cerebrovascular accidents, or limb-threatening gangrene of the extremities). In many cases, these dramatic acute manifestations are the patient's first sign of the presence of the atherosclerotic lesion, which evolved silently over decades.

What mechanisms may explain this often dramatic transition from chronic to acute manifestations of human atherosclerosis? Why does a lesion that has remained silent for many years suddenly produce such dramatic manifestations? Several possible explanations have been advanced including thrombosis with or without plaque rupture, vasospasm, and hemorrhage into a plaque. Each of these mechanisms may singly or in concert explain the rapid shift from the chronic to the acute phase of atherosclerotic disease. We have considered already how immune and inflammatory mechanisms may contribute to lesion initiation and evolution. Might similar phenomena contribute to unleashing the pathogenic mechanisms listed above?

REGULATION OF LOCAL HEMOCOMPATIBILITY BY INFLAMMATORY MEDIATORS

In ordinary circumstances the vascular endothelium is one of the few surfaces, natural or synthetic, that can maintain blood in a liquid state. This property, denoted hemocompatibility, results from a variety of antithrombotic, anti-coagulant, and fibrinolytic properties of the normal endothelial surface (53,54). For example, endothelial cells can synthesize the antithrombotic arachidonate metabolite prostacyclin (55). These cells also can synthesize heparin sulfate molecules that interact with antithrombin III to furnish a natural anticoagulant interface between the arterial wall and blood (56). Endothelial cells also can express thrombomodulin, a key element in regulation of the protein S and protein C anticoagulant pathways (54).

Endothelial cells also can express functions that promote hemostasis providing mechanisms that can limit hemorrhage after arterial injury. Examples include synthesis of inhibitors of plasminogen activator, von Willebrand factor (important for adherence of platelets), and a tissue factor-like procoagulant activity. The *in vivo* significance of the tissue factor expression, demonstrated in culture cells, remains controversial. Nonetheless, it is clear that the ability of the luminal endothelial cells to maintain blood in a liquid state depends on a dynamic balance of anticoagulant, antithrombotic, and fibrinolytic pathways on the one hand and procoagulant, antifibrinolytic, and prothrombotic capacities on the other. The key factors that govern this hemostatic balance of the endothelial surface appear to be cytokine mediators of the inflammatory and immune responses. In studies of cultured endothelial cells, IL-1 and TNF potently regulate most of these properties that determine blood compatibility in a manner that favors hemostasis (57–60). In the atheroma, the source of the regulatory cytokines could be activated mononuclear phagocytes, cells which abound in these lesions. An additional local source of IL-1 and perhaps TNF could be intrinsic blood vessel wall cells themselves, notably smooth muscle (10,61). These locally produced cytokines may well contribute to the alterations in regional hemostasis that unleash the acute syndromes of arterial occlusive disease.

REGULATION OF VASCULAR TONE BY CYTOKINES

Vasospasm might contribute also to sudden interruption in blood flow by occluding points of stenosis by a fixed lesion or by promoting stasis, one of Virchow's classic triad of factors promoting thrombosis. IL-1 increases the production by endothelial cells of platelet-activating factor, a potent coronary vasoconstrictor (62). IL-1 also stimulates arachidonate metabolism in target tissues. Each cell type exhibits its own particular pattern of prostaglandin synthesis. In the case of endothelium, IL-1 stimulates the production of prostacyclin, a vasodilator and antithrombotic product of the arachidonate cascade (55). However, in numerically more abundant smooth muscle cells, the production of prostaglandin E_2 by IL-1 far exceeds that of prostacyclin (11). Prostaglandin E_2 and $F_{2\alpha}$, the major products of IL-1-stimulated human smooth muscle cell arachidonate metabolism, contract coronary arteries. Interleukin-1 can augment endothelial production of the potent coronary vasoconstrictor endothelin (63) also. These findings illustrate how regional release of vasoconstrictor prostanoids or peptides provoked by inflammatory cytokines could promote local coronary vasospasm.

PARTICIPATION OF CYTOKINES IN MICROVASCULAR HEMORRHAGE WITHIN A PLAQUE AS A CAUSE OF SUDDEN LESION EXPANSION

An alternative explanation for the sudden occlusions that complicate chronic atherosclerotic lesions is hemorrhage into the plaque. The mass effect could expand rapidly a nonobstructing lesion to a total occlusion. The pathophysiology of such intraplaque bleeds may involve the extensive neovascular channels of atherosclerotic plaques, a phenomenon noted many years ago, but recently the focus of renewed attention (64). Such new blood vessels may exhibit increased fragility, in analogy to those found in diabetic retinopathy. How could inflammatory mediators contribute to neovascularization? The role of macrophages in neoangiogenesis has been appreciated for some time (65), a finding that suggests that monokines such as TNF or IL-1 might account for some of the angiogenic activity produced by activated mononuclear phagocytes. Indeed, a number of groups recently have demonstrated that administration of recombinant TNF can promote new vessel formation in standard angiogenesis assay preparations (66). Whether these effects are direct or indirect are uncertain, yet these findings indicate that locally produced monokines may contribute to the formation of new blood vessels within atheromata that form the substrate for intraplaque hemorrhage.

CONCLUSIONS

Despite the prevalence and clinical significance of arteriosclerosis, the pathogenic mechanisms have remained controversial. Some consider alterations in plasma lipoproteins the prime pathogenic factor in development of atheroma. In some circumstances, however, plaque formation may not require the participation of lipids (67). We favor a more synoptic view of human atherogenesis. Numerous factors doubtless contribute to the formation of these lesions. In some cases alterations in lipoprotein metabolism may be primary; in others alternative mechanisms may come into play, possibly including viral infections, immune complex deposition, the response to ionizing radiation, and metabolic diseases (e.g., homocysteinuria, pseudoxanthoma elasticum, and the "collagen vascular diseases").

We advocate the viewpoint that common pathogenic mechanisms operate during lesion formation, evolution, and the transition from chronic to acute disease regardless of the triggering and contributory mechanisms at play in each individual. In each phase of the life history of an atherosclerotic lesion, we believe that mediators of the immune and inflammatory response such as the cytokines IL-1 and TNF may influence their development. Many of these hypotheses are based on observations with cultured cells. These ideas are currently susceptible to investigation in animal preparations. However valuable, such experimental approaches are limited as none mimics human atherogenesis perfectly. Future investigations must test the relevance of these hypotheses to the human lesion *in situ*. If the cytokines do play pathogenic roles in human atherosclerosis, they may provide a target for therapeutic intervention in the future. Selective antagonists that block the effects of cytokines conceivably could prove beneficial. In any case, successful efforts to prevent, slow, or reverse human atherogenesis will require continued appreciation for the cellular and molecular mechanisms that underlie this process.

ACKNOWLEDGMENTS

I thank my co-workers and collaborators who have contributed to the studies from my laboratory referred to here. Those studies were supported by Grant HL-34636, the American Heart Association, Massachusetts Affiliate, and in part with facilities and funds provided by the U.S. Department of Agriculture, Agricultural Research Service to Tufts University under contract number 53-3K06-5-10. Dr. Libby is an Established Investigator of the American Heart Association.

REFERENCES

1. Munro JM, Cotran RS. The pathogenesis of atherosclerosis: atherogenesis and inflammation. *Lab Invest* 1988;58:249–261.
2. Hansson GK, Jonasson L, Seifert PS, Stemme S. Immune mechanisms in atherosclerosis. *Arteriosclerosis* 1989;9:567–578.
3. Libby P. The active roles of cells of the blood vessel wall in health and disease. *Mol Aspects Med* 1987;9:499–567.
4. Aqel NM, Ball RY, Waldmann H, Mitchinson MJ. Identification of macrophages and smooth muscle cells in human atherosclerosis using monoclonal antibodies. *J Pathol* 1985;146:197–204.
5. Klurfeld DM. Identification of foam cells in human atherosclerotic lesions as macrophages using monoclonal antibodies. *Arch Pathol Lab Med* 1985;109:445–449.
6. Jonasson L, Holm J, Skalli O, Bonders G, Hansson GK. Regional accumulations of T cells, macrophages, and smooth muscle cells in the human atherosclerotic plaque. *Arteriosclerosis* 1986;6:131–138.
7. Gown AM, Tsukada T, Ross R. Human atherosclerosis II. Immunocytochemical analysis of the cellular composition of human atherosclerotic lesions. *Am J Pathol* 1986;125:191–207.
8. Emeson EE, Robertson AL Jr. T-lymphocytes in aortic and coronary intimas. *Am J Pathol* 1988;130:369–376.
9. Loppnow H, Libby P. Comparative analysis of cytokine induction in human vascular endothelial and smooth muscle cells. *Lymphokine Res* 1989;8:293–299.
10. Warner SJC, Libby P. Human vascular smooth muscle cells: target for and source of tumor necrosis factor. *J Immunol* 1989;142:100–109.

11. Libby P, Warner SJC, Friedman GB. Interleukin-1: a mitogen for human vascular smooth muscle cells that induces the release of growth-inhibitory prostanoids. *J Clin Invest* 1988;88: 487–498.

12. Raines EW, Dower SK, Ross R. Interleukin-1 mitogenic activity for fibroblasts and smooth muscle cells is due to PDGF-AA. *Science* 1989;243:393–396.

13. Libby P, Friedman GB, Salomon RN. Cytokines as modulators of cell proliferation in fibrotic diseases. *Am Rev Respir Dis* 1989;140:1114–1117.

14. Brown MS, Goldstein JL. Lipoprotein metabolism in the macrophage: implications for cholesterol deposition in atherosclerosis. *Annu Rev Biochem* 1983;52:223–261.

15. Steinberg D, Parthasarathy S, Carew TE, Khoo JC, Witztum JL. Beyond cholesterol. Modifications of low-density lipoprotein that increase its atherogenicity. *N Engl J Med* 1989;320:915–924.

16. Stary HC. Macrophages, macrophage foam cells, and eccentric intimal thickening in the coronary arteries of young children. *Atherosclerosis* 1987;64:91–108.

17. Komatsu A, Wissler RW, Vesselinovitch D. Cell populations in atheromatous lesions in young people [Abstract]. *Circulation* 1989;80(No. 4):II-332.

18. Stary HC. Evolution and progression of atherosclerotic lesions in coronary arteries of children and young adults. *Arteriosclerosis* 1989;9(Suppl I):I-19–I-32.

19. Jokinen MP, Clarkson TB, Pritchard RW. Animal models in atherosclerosis research. *Exp Mol Pathol* 1985;42:1–28.

20. Poole JCF, Florey HW. Changes in the endothelium of the aorta and the behavior of macrophages in experimental atheroma of rabbits. *J Pathol Bacteriol* 1958;75:245–253.

21. Gerrity RG, Naito HK, Richardson M, Schwartz CJ. Dietary induced atherogenesis in swine: Morphology of the intima in prelesion stages. *Am J Pathol* 1979;95:775–786.

22. Joris T, Nunnari JJ, Krolikowski FJ, Majno G. Studies on the pathogenesis of atherosclerosis. I. Adhesion and emigration of mononuclear cells in the aorta of hypercholesterolemic rats. *Am J Pathol* 1983;113:341–358.

23. Faggioto A, Ross R, Harker L. Studies of hypercholesterolemia in the nonhuman primate. I. Changes that lead to fatty streak formation. *Arteriosclerosis* 1984;4:323–340.

24. Majno G, Zand T, Nunnari JJ, Kowala MC, Joris I. Intimal responses to shear stress, hypercholesterolemia, and hypertension. Studies in the rat aorta. In: Simionescu N, Simionescu M, eds. *Endothelial cell biology.* New York: Plenum Publishing Corporation. 1988:349–367.

25. Lansman JB, Hallam TJ, Rink TJ. Single stretch-activated ion channels in vascular endothelial cells as mechanotransducers. *Nature* 1987;325:811–813.

26. Lansman JB. Endothelial mechanosensors—going with the flow. *Nature* 1988;331:481–482.

27. Olesen SP, Clapham DE, Davies PF. Haemodynamic shear stress activates a K+ current in vascular endothelial cells. *Nature* 1988;331:168–170.

28. Bevilacqua MP, Pober JS, Majeau GR, Cotran RS, Gimbrone MA Jr. Interleukin-1 acts on cultured human vascular endothelium to increase the adhesion of polymorphonuclear leukocytes, monocytes and related leukocyte cell lines. *J Clin Invest* 1985;76:2003–2011.

29. Dustin ML, Rothlein R, Bhan AK, Dinarello CA, Springer TA. Induction by IL-1 and interferon-gamma: tissue distribution, biochemistry, and function of a natural adherence molecule (ICAM-1). *J Immunol* 1986;137:245–254.

30. Pohlman TH, Stanness KA, Beatty PG, Ochs HD, Harlan JM. An endothelial cell surface factor(s) induced in vitro by lipopolysaccharide, interleukin 1, and tumor necrosis factor-alpha increases neutrophil adherence by a CDw 18-dependent mechanism. *J Immunol* 1986;136: 4548–4553.

31. Aronson FR, Libby P, Brandon EP, Janicka MW, Mier JW. Interleukin-2 rapidly induces natural killer cell adhesion to human endothelial cells: a potential mechanism for endothelial injury. *J Immunol* 1988;141:158–163.

32. Bevilacqua MP, Stengelin S, Gimbrone MA Jr, Seed B. Endothelial leukocyte adhesion molecule 1: an inducible receptor for neutrophils related to complement regulatory proteins and lectins. *Science* 1989;243:1160–1165.

33. McEver RP, Beckstead JH, Moore KL, Marshall-Carlson L, Bainton DF. GMP-140, a platelet alpha-granule membrane protein, is also synthesized by vascular endothelial cells and is localized in Weibel-Palade bodies. *J Clin Invest* 1989;84:92–99.

34. Larsen E, Celi A, Gilbert GE, et al. PADGEM protein: a receptor that mediates the interaction of activated platelets with neutrophils and monocytes. *Cell* 1989;59:305–312.

35. Valente AJ, Fowler SR, Sprague EA, Kelley JL, Suenram CA, Schwartz CJ. Initial characterization of a peripheral blood mononuclear cell chemoattractant derived from cultured arterial smooth muscle cells. *Am J Pathol* 1984;117:409–417.
36. Mazzone T, Jensen M, Chait A. Human arterial wall cells secrete factors that are chemotactic for monocytes. *Proc Natl Acad Sci USA* 1983;80:5094–5097.
37. Graves DT, Jiang YL, Williamson MJ, Valente AJ. Identification of monocyte chemotactic activity produced by malignant cells. *Science* 1989;245:1490–1493.
38. Yoshimura T, Yuhki N, Moore SK, Appella E, Lerman MI, Leonard EJ. Human monocyte chemoattractant protein-1 (MCP-1). Full-length cDNA cloning, expression in mitogen-stimulated blood mononuclear leukocytes, and sequence similarity to mouse competence gene JE. *FEBS Lett* 1989;244:487–493.
39. Sica A, Wang JM, Colotta F, et al. Monocyte chemotactic and activating factor gene expression induced in endothelial cells by IL-1 and TNF. *J Immunol* (in press).
40. Rosenfeld ME, Tsukada T, Chait A, Bierman EL, Gown AM, Ross R. Fatty streak expansion and maturation in watanabe heritable hyperlipemic and comparably hyperchlolesterolemic fat-fed rabbits. *Arterioclerosis* 1987;7:24–34.
41. Rosenfeld ME, Tsukada T, Gown AM, Ross R. Fatty streak initiation in watanabe heritable hyperlipemic and comparably hypercholesterolemic fat-fed rabbits. *Arteriosclerosis* 1987;7:9–23.
42. Koo C, Wernette-Hammond ME, Garcia Z, et al. Uptake of cholesterol-rich remnant lipoproteins by human monocyte-derived macrophages is mediated by low density lipoprotein receptors. *J Clin Invest* 1988;81:1332–1340.
43. Kodama T, Rohrer L, Freeman M, Krieger M. Binding properties of a purified acetyl-LDL receptor. *Circulation* 1989;80:II-333.
44. Shimokado K, Raines EW, Madtes DK, Barrett TB, Benditt EP, Ross R. A significant part of macrophage-derived growth factor consists of at least two forms of PDGF. *Cell* 1985;43:277–286.
45. Martinet Y, Bitterman PB, Mornex JF, Grotendorst GR, Martin GR, Crystal RG. Activated human monocytes express the c-sis proto-oncogene and release a mediator showing PDGF-like activity. *Nature* 1986;319:158–160.
46. Madtes DK, Raines EW, Sakariassen KS, et al. Induction of transforming growth factor-alpha in activated human alveolar macrophages. *Cell* 1988;53:285–293.
47. Jonasson L, Holm J, Skalli O, Gabbiani G, Hansson GK. Expression of class II transplantation antigen on vascular smooth muscle cells in human atherosclerosis. *J Clin Invest* 1985;76:125–131.
48. Hansson GK, Jonasson L, Holm J, Claesson-Welsh L. Class II MHC antigen expression in the atherosclerotic plaque: smooth muscle cells express HLA-DR, HLA-DQ and the invariant gamma chain. *Clin Exp Immunol* 1986;64:261–268.
49. Pober JS, Collins T, Gimbrone MA Jr, Libby P, Reiss CS. Inducible expression of class II major histocompatibility complex antigens and the immunogenicity of vascular endothelium. *Transplantation* 1986;41:141–146.
50. Hansson GK, Jonasson L, Holm J, Clowes MK, Clowes A. Gamma interferon regulates vascular smooth muscle proliferation and Ia expression in vivo and in vitro. *Circ Res* 1988;63:712–719.
51. Warner SJC, Friedman GB, Libby P. Regulation of major histocompatibility gene expression in cultured human vascular smooth muscle cells. *Arteriosclerosis* 1989;9:279–288.
52. Hansson GK, Holm J, Jonasson L. Detection of activated T lymphocytes in the human atherosclerotic plaque. *Am J Pathol* 1989;135(1):169–175.
53. Gimbrone MA Jr. ed. *Vascular endothelium in hemostasis and thrombosis* Edinburgh: Churchill Livingstone, 1986:250 pp.
54. Esmon CT. The regulation of natural anticoagulant pathways. *Science* 1987;235:1348–1352.
55. Weksler BB, Marcus AJ, Jaffe EA. Synthesis of prostaglandin I_2 (prostacyclin) by cultured human and bovine endothelial cells. *Proc Natl Acad Sci USA* 1977;74:3922–3926.
56. Marcum JA, Rosenberg RD. Heparin-like molecules with anticoagulant activity are synthesized by cultured endothelial cells. *Biochem Biophy Res Comm* 1985;126:365–372.
57. Bevilacqua MP, Pober JS, Majeau GR, Cotran RS, Gimbrone MA Jr. Interleukin-1 (IL-1) induces biosynthesis and cell surface expression of procoagulant activity in human vascular endothelial cells. *J Exp Med* 1984;160:618–623.

58. Bevilacqua MP, Schleef R, Gimbrone MA Jr, Loskutoff DJ. Regulation of the fibrinolytic system of cultured human vascular endothelium by IL-1. *J Clin Invest* 1986;78:587–591.
59. Stern DM, Bank I, Nawroth PP, et al. Self-regulation of procoagulant events on the endothelial cell surface. *J Exp Med* 1985;162:1223–1235.
60. Nachman RL, Hajjar KA, Silverstein RL, Dinarello CA. Interleukin 1 induces endothelial cell synthesis of plasminogen activator inhibitor. *J Exp Med* 1986;163:1595–1600.
61. Libby P, Ordovas JM, Birinyi LK, Auger KR, Dinarello CA. Inducible interleukin-1 expression in human vascular smooth muscle cells. *J Clin Invest* 1986;78:1432–1438.
62. Bussolino F, Breviario F, Tetta C, Aglietta M, Mantovani A, Dejana E. Interleukin 1 stimulates platelet-activating factor production in cultured human endothelial cells. *J Clin Invest* 1986;77:2027–2033.
63. Yoshizumi M, Kurihara H, Morita T, et al. Interleukin 1 increases the production of endothelin by cultured endothelial cells. *Circulation* 1989;80:II-5.
64. Barger A, Beeuwkes IR, Lainey L, Silverman K. Hypothesis: vasa vasorum and neovascularization of human coronary arteries. *N Engl J Med* 1984;310:175–177.
65. Polverini PJ, Cotran RS, Gimbrone MA Jr, Unanue ER. Activated macrophages induce vascular proliferation. *Nature* 1977;269:804–806.
66. Leibovich S, Polverini P, Shipard H, Wiseman D, Shiveley V, Nuseir N. Macrophage-induced angiogenesis is mediated by tumor necrosis factor. *Nature* 1987;329:630–632.
67. Libby P, Salomon RN, Payne DD, Schoen FJ, Pober JS. Functions of vascular wall cells related to the development of transplantation-associated coronary arteriosclerosis. *Transplant Proc* 1989;21:3677–3684.

Atherosclerosis Reviews, Volume 21,
edited by A. Leaf and P. C. Weber.
Raven Press, Ltd., New York © 1990.

Atherosclerosis Risk Factor Modification by n-3 Fatty Acids

Peter C. Weber

Universität München, Institut für Prophylaxe und Epidemiologie der Kreislaufkrankheiten, 8000 München 2, Federal Republic of Germany

Atherosclerosis, the most prominent cause of morbidity and mortality in Western populations, is a multifactorial disease. Table 1 shows that both genetic and exogenous factors are involved in its pathogenesis and clinical course. Activation of platelets, monocytes, and neutrophils, and the coagulations cascade at sites of endothelial injury are characteristic of early events in the pathogenesis of atherosclerosis (1).

This brief review addresses the potential role of n-3 polyunsaturated fatty acids (PUFAs) in modifying key cellular events in the atherosclerotic process, that is the function of platelets, monocytes/macrophages, and endothelial and vascular smooth muscle cells.

EICOSANOIDS AS MODULATORS OF CELL FUNCTION

Eicosanoids, the oxygenated metabolites of arachidonic acid C20:4n-6 (AA) and related 20-carbon PUFAs modulate a wide variety of physiologic and pathologic cellular reactions (2-4). The position of the eicosanoids in modulating cell stimulus-response coupling and in mediating cell-to-cell communication is schematically shown in Fig. 1.

All eicosanoids are derived from PUFAs, which must be provided in the diet (5). Formation and function of eicosanoids is controlled by the specific cell stimulus and at the level of uptake, release, and oxygenation of the precursor fatty acids. Some eicosanoids, such as thromboxane (TX) A2 and leukotriene (LT) B4, may amplify an initial (Ca^{2+}-related) signal of cell activation by stimulating specific membrane receptors coupled to the activation of phospholipases, thereby increasing intracellular Ca^{2+}-concentration further. Other eicosanoids, such as prostaglandin (PG) I_2, might blunt—via increasing cAMP-levels—an initial signal for cell activation by decreasing intracellular Ca^{2+} concentrations.

In our Western dietary conditions, AA is by far the dominant eicosanoid precursor fatty acid. Compatible with the significant role of this system in common "Western" diseases is the fact that interference with eicosanoid formation

TABLE 1. *Risk factors of atherosclerosis and mechanisms involved*

Nonmodifiable factors	Modifiable factors	Mechanisms
Family history	Inadequate nutrition	Fatty acids
Male sex	Hyperlipidemia	Eicosanoids
Age	Obesity	Platelets
	Diabetes mellitus	Monocytes/macrophages
	Hypertension	Endothelial cells
	Cigarette smoking	Smooth muscle cells
	Physical inactivity	Growth factors
		Cytokines
		Cholesterol/modified cholesterol
		Foam cells
		Coagulation factors

or action is a characteristic feature of potent antiplatelet and other cardiovascular drugs, steroidal and nonsteroidal antiinflammatory and antiproliferative compounds (6) (Table 2). A change of eicosanoid formation and eicosanoid-dependent, pathological cellular reactions may be achieved also by a nutritional modification of the eicosanoid precursor fatty acid pool (5). In Table 3, approximate numbers of the frequency of CHD in three populations and the characteristic differences in the content of AA and eicosapentaenoic acid, C20:5n-3

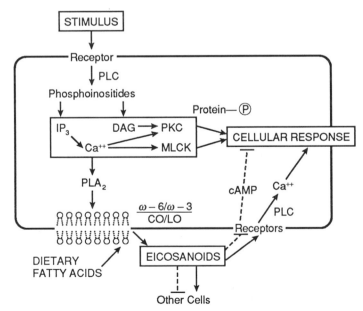

FIG. 1. Scheme of the putative role of n-6 and n-3 eicosanoid precursor fatty acids in membrane phospholipids as determined by dietary intake and their eicosanoids for the modulation of stimulus-response coupling and cell-to-cell communication. PLC, phospholipase C; IP_3, inositol trisphosphate; DAG, 1,2 diacylglycerol; PKC, proteinkinase C; MLCK, myosin light-chain kinase; PLA_2, phospholipase A_2; Co, cyclooxygenase; LO, lipoxygenase; Protein-P, phosphorylated protein.

TABLE 2. *Drugs used in atherothrombotic cardiovascular disorders*

Antiplatelet drugs
Anticoagulants
Antihypertensives
Lipid-lowering drugs
Fibrinolytic drugs
Antianginal drugs; EDRF-related
Calcium antagonists

Note: n-3 fatty acids act at similar sites where these drugs act.

(EPA) in membrane phospholipids, illustrate this intriguing relationship (5,7–13). In fact, with the adoption of Western dietary habits, leading to an increase in fat intake and a relative reduction of n-3 fatty acid content in their diet, Japanese have experienced increasing mortality rates from coronary heart disease (CHD) (14).

ORIGIN AND INTERRELATIONSHIP OF n-6 AND n-3 FATTY ACIDS

In the mammalian organism, fatty acids belonging to different families such as the n-3 and the n-6 fatty acids cannot be formed *de novo* or interconverted. Therefore, nutritional intake determines to a great extent the fatty acid composition of phospholipids in plasma and in cell membranes (Fig. 2) (15).

Linoleic acid (C18:2n-6) of plant origin, and the parent fatty acid of the n-6 fatty acid family, is desaturated and elongated to AA in animals and in humans. Through its conversion to TX, AA is a potent aggregator of platelets (2). After infusion or dietary intake of AA, *in vivo* animal (16) and human (17) studies show that platelets are more sticky and lead to thrombus formation. In contrast to AA and EPA, C20:3n-3 does not aggregate platelets *in vitro* (9,15,18). After dietary intake, it reduces platelet aggregation *ex vivo* (18–20).

The n-3 fatty acids in the diet are absorbed rapidly and are incorporated into plasma phospholipids (21), where they replace arachidonic acids. At the same

TABLE 3. *AA, EPA, and frequency of death from coronary heart disease (CHD) in three populations[a]*

	Platelet phospholipid fatty acids[b]		Ratio n-6:n-3	CHD (% death)
Europe, USA	20 to 26	0.1 to 0.7	50	40
Japan	18 to 22	$\approx$1.0 to 2.5	12	12
Greenland Eskimo	8.3 to 9.0	6.4 to 8.0	1.2	7

Note: Data from refs. 7 to 10, 12 to 14, 18 to 21 and 51.
[a] All values are approximate.
[b] AA (C20:4n-6) and EPA (C20:5n-3).

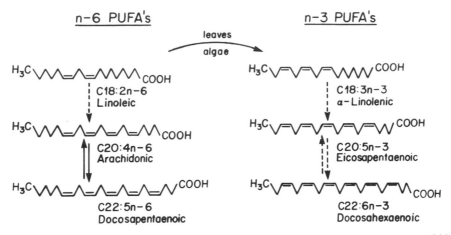

FIG. 2. Origin and metabolism of n-6 and n-3 polyunsaturated fatty acids, arachidonic acid (C20: 4n-6) and eicosapentaenoic acid (C20:5n-3).

time, arachidonic acid is redistributed partly to the triacylglacerol or cholesterol ester fractions (22). Most of the incorporation of n-3 fatty acids into cellular membrane phospholipids appears to occur during cell formation, at least under *in vivo* conditions in the unstimulated cell (21). Also it seems that in the adult human organism *in vivo*, the formation of the 20-carbon atom eicosanoid precursor fatty acids from their respective short-chain parent fatty acids, C18:2n-6 or C18:3n-3, is of limited capacity (21). This implies that in humans the long-chain eicosanoid precursor fatty acids in the diet might have a more direct effect on the eicosanoid precursor pool than do their C18 parent fatty acids.

MECHANISM OF ACTION OF DIETARY n-3 FATTY ACIDS

In an early study (20), we found that it is possible to induce less-reactive platelets and reduced formation of proaggregatory and vasoconstrictive thromboxane in Caucasians by substituting mackerel-rich n-3 PUFAs as the sole source of dietary fat. In plasma and platelet membrane phospholipids, n-3 fatty acids increased at the expense of AA and other n-6 unsaturated fatty acids, thereby inducing a pattern of fatty acids similar to that found in Greenland Eskimos and in Japanese. It was characterized by a low content of AA and high contents of EPA and docosahexaenoic acid (DHA) (Tables 3 and 4).

In subsequent studies (18,19), the Western diet was supplemented with 10 to 40 ml/day of cod liver oil (CLO) providing about 1 to 4 g of EPA and about 1 to 5 g of DHA per day. The studies showed that EPA and DHA were time- and dose-dependently incorporated into plasma, platelet, and erythrocyte membrane phospholipids at the expense of the n-6 PUFAs, C20:4n-6 and C18:2n-6. Bleeding time increased; platelet count, platelet aggregation (adenosine diphos-

TABLE 4. *Dietary modification of platelet phospholipid fatty acids*

	Platelet	Phospholipid	Fatty acids (%)	
	18:2n-6	20:4n-6	20:5n-3[b]	22:6n-3[b]
Control (Western) diet	9	26	0.4	2.3
Cod liver oil				
10 ml, 4 weeks	8	23	1.3[a]	3.0
20 ml, 4 weeks	7	22[a]	2.5[a]	4.1
40 ml, 4 weeks	7	20[a]	4.6[a]	5.5[a]
300 to 600 g/day, 6 days	5[a]	18[a]	5.0[a]	6.0[a]

Note: Data adapted from refs. 18 to 20.
[a] $p < 0.05$ vs control diet.
[b] n-3 fatty acids (EPA + DHA) ranges from 2 to 15 g/day.

phate), collagen, and associated thromboxane formation decreased. Blood pressure and pressure responses to norepinephrine and angiotensin II fell, without major changes in plasma catecholamines and red cell cation fluxes, but slight decreases were found in renin, urinary aldosterone, kallikrein and PG E_2 and F_{2a}. Biochemical and functional changes were rapid at onset, but reversed 4 to 6 weeks after cessation of the fish oil supplement (18,19).

In an attempt to explain functional effects of a dietary shift from the n-6 to the n-3 PUFA on the basis of an alteration in the spectrum of eicosanoids produced, the spectrum of eicosanoids after manipulation of the dietary supply with n-6 or n-3 fatty acids has been analyzed (25). The experiments were performed after dietary substitution (mackerel for 1 to 7 days) or supplementation (fish oil for 1 to 5 months, corresponding to 2.5 to 11 g EPA + DHA/day) of the western diet in male Europeans (23,24).

After consumption of dietary fish or fish oil rich in the n-3 PUFA, EPA and DHA tests indicated that TXB_3 was formed from EPA in stimulated platelets at only 5% to 15% that of TXB_2, which, itself, was reduced to 30% to 50% of the control (15,26). In volunteers with high basal excretion rates of the major TX metabolite (TXB_2-M), the excretion of $TXB_{2/3}$-M was reduced to normal after the n-3 PUFA-enriched diet (19).

Importantly, and in contrast to the pattern of TX formation, PGI3-M increased dose- and time-dependently up to 50% of an *unchanged* PGI_2-M excretion (19,24). PGI_2-M excretion even increased when mackerel was substituted in the Western diet (24).

After dietary supplementation of n-3 fatty acids, peripheral white blood cells formed LTB_5 from incorporated cellular EPA after stimulation with Ca^{2+} ionophore A23187 (26). The conversion rates of cellular EPA and AA to LTB_5 + LTB_4, respectively, were similar. The products formed were related quantitatively to their parent fatty acids in the cellular lipids. At high concentrations of exogenous EPA, the formation of the highly chemotactic LTB_4 from endogenous AA was suppressed to a large extent. In similar long-term supplementation experiments, the formation of LTB_4 also fell, and granulocyte and monocyte function was inhibited (27).

CELLULAR AND FATTY ACID SPECIFICITIES

Differences exist in the ways various cell types (neutrophils, platelets, and endothelial cells) incorporate and/or metabolize n-3 and n-6 fatty acids, which are provided in the diet, to eicosanoids. Differences exist also between the n-3 and n-6 fatty acids incorporated into specific cellular phopholipid subclasses: e.g., *in vivo* the long-chain n-3 fatty acids seem to be incorporated only to an insignificant extent in phosphatidyl-inositol (28). However, they are incorporated in phosphatidyl-choline and phosphatidyl-ethanolamine and in alkylacyl-glycerophosphocholine. This might have important implications for cell function because in addition to different eicosanoid precursors, different molecular species of other lipid mediators, such as diglycerides and platelet-activating factor precursors (29–31) with different biological functions might be formed.

Using ethyl-esters of the purified fatty acids, EPA and DHA, which are major constituents of fish oils, antiplatelet effects of both compounds were demonstrated recently (21). In the same study, dietary DHA was shown to be retroconverted to EPA and to be metabolized to PGI3 (32). PGI3-M was detectable within 4 hr after a single dose of DHA. Therefore, DHA may reduce platelet aggregability both by a mechanism related to formation of PGI3 and by a direct effect on platelet function related to alterations in membrane composition.

In summary, dietary EPA + DHA, which partially replace AA and linoleic acid in a specific time- and dose-dependent manner in plasma and certain cellular phospholipid subclasses, induce a series of biochemical events. Once incorporated in cellular membranes, DHA seems to be released upon cell stimulation less readily (33), reducing substrate availability for eicosanoid generation and decreasing potent amplification mechanisms to which AA metabolites contribute, e.g., as a cellular response to injury (34).

In addition to reducing levels of AA and most of its eicosanoid derivatives (with the exception of PGI_2), the n-3 fatty acids EPA and also DHA, which can be retroconverted to EPA, serve as precursors to a class of eicosanoids having an attenuated and desirable spectrum of biological activity with respect to platelet aggregation, and white blood cell- and vascular function (26). Kinetic and dose-response studies in healthy volunteers indicate that changes in plasma fatty acid spectra and eicosanoid formation occur rapidly within hours, are demonstrable for the entire supplementation period, and are dose related to the amounts of n-3 PUFA provided in the diet. The changes in cellular fatty acid composition occur during cell formation and are demonstrable for several weeks even after cessation of the dietary supply with n-3 PUFA. This indicates a biologically important relationship. Furthermore, it suggests that in addition to the membrane phospholipid fatty acid pool for eicosanoid formation, there is obviously another, rapidly available metabolic pool of eicosanoid precursors which is related more directly to dietary intake and probably not dependent upon release of fatty acids from membrane phospholipids.

OTHER BIOCHEMICAL AND FUNCTIONAL EFFECTS OF n-3 FATTY ACIDS

Meanwhile, a variety of additional effects of n-3 fatty acids have been described, including those that are summarized in Table 5. Basically, these effects are the result of modifications of the fatty acid composition of cell membranes and critical lipid pools where n-6 and n-3 fatty acids and their mediators obviously fulfill important and diverse physiological functions. Besides their effects on the eicosanoid system, n-3 fatty acids reduce the formation of platelet-activating factor, PAF (35), a proinflammatory and proaggregatory lipid mediator of potential importance in atherosclerosis (35).

Significant reductions of vascular intimal hyperplasia in autologous arteriovenous grafts (36) and of injury and elevated cholesterol-induced atherosclerosis have been reported in animal experiments after feeding fish oils rich in n-3 fatty acids (37,38). These antiatherosclerotic effects of n-3 fatty acids might be due to several mechanisms, including modifications of the AA cascade, reduction of PAF formation, inhibition of the coagulation potential (39), and, importantly, the reduction in synthesis and action of peptide mediators of cell proliferation including interleukin-1 (Il-1), and tumor necrosis factor (TNF) (40) as well as the platelet-derived growth factor, PDGF (41), which all have been

TABLE 5. *Summary of biochemical and functional effects of n-3 fatty acids that might be relevant for their antiatherosclerotic action*

n-3 fatty acids reduce risk/precipitating factors	n-3 fatty acids increase protective factors
Arachidonic acid	
Platelet aggregation	Prostacyclin formation
Thromboxane formation	PGI_2 + PGI_3
PDGF synthesis	
Monocyte/macrophage function	Endothelial-dependent
Leukotriene formation	Vasorelaxation, EDRF
PAF formation	
IL-1 and TNF production	Fibrinolytic activity
Oxygen-free radicals	
Blood pressure/BP response	Red-cell deformability
VLDL, triglycerides	Vascular compliance
LDL-size	
Fibrinogen	
Intimal hyperplasia	
Blood viscosity	

Note: VLDL, very-low-density lipoprotein.

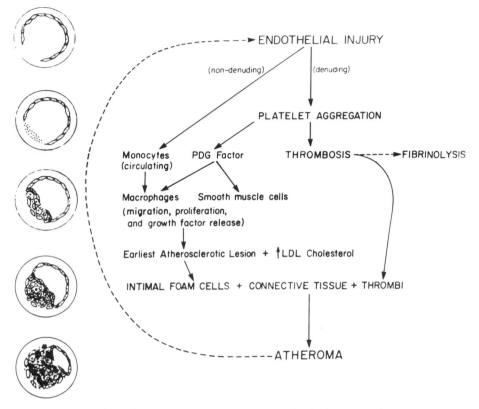

FIG. 3. Sequential steps in the pathogenesis of atherosclerosis.

found recently after n-3 fatty acids. These effects and the potential of n-3 fatty acids to increase the formation/release of endothelial-derived relaxation factor (EDRF) (42), to increase erythrocyte deformability, and to reduce blood viscosity (43) also may improve organ perfusion and increase arterial compliance (44).

Altogether, these studies indicate that n-3 fatty acids have the potential to interfere at several steps with the atheroclerotic precess as depicted in Fig. 3.

DIETARY n-3 FATTY ACIDS AND PREVENTION OF ATHEROSCLEROSIS?

We do not know at present the biological significance and the cause of the fact that AA constitutes by far the major precursor fatty acid of eicosanoids and related lipid mediators under our Western dietary conditions. One reason might be the increasingly uniform supply of n-6 fatty acids in our food chain, i.e., in vegetable oils and in livestock fattened with grain rich in C18:2n-6, which in the

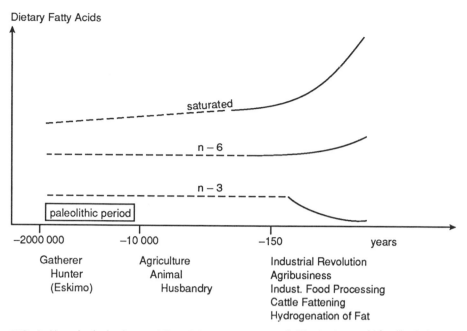

FIG. 4. Hypothetical scheme of the relative percentages of different fatty acid families in human nutrition as extrapolated from cross-sectional analyses of contemporary hunter-gatherer populations and from longitudinal observations and their putative changes during the preceding 150 years. Adapted from ref. 55.

mammalian organism is slowly desaturated and elongated to AA. According to a recent review, this might not have been always the case (45). Irrespective of whether the putative diet of our remote ancestors was based more on animal or on vegetable sources, their nutrition probably was lower in fat and relatively rich in n-3 fatty acids (45). A scheme of these relationships and their hypothetical change over time is depicted in Fig. 4.

Longitudinal as well as transcultural studies point to a currently low intake of n-3 fatty acids as a characteristic feature of "Western" nutrition when compared to contemporary nonwestern, historic, and prehistoric controls.

So far, published data of controlled trials incorporating clinical end points with regard to n-3 PUFA are encouraging: In 3 of 5 published prospective studies, n-3 PUFA were effective in reducing restenosis after percutaneous transluminal coronary angioplasty (45–49). Three retrospective epidemiological studies, evaluating the correlation between fish intake and mortality from CHD demonstrated a significant inverse relationship between fish consumption and coronary heart disease (50–53), corroborating observation in Greenland Eskimos (7,10) and in Japanese (11–13). Importantly, in a recently published, large, controlled, prospective trial on dietary intervention in 2,033 men who had recovered from myocardial infarction, those subjects advised to eat fatty fish had a 29% reduction in a 2-year all-cause mortality ($p < 0.05$) compared with those who were not so advised (54). The advice on fat reduction plus an increase of the polyunsaturated/saturated fatty acid ratio, or the advice to increase fiber intake were ineffective in this trial. This study is the first prospective dietary intervention trial for secondary prevention of CHD that demonstrates clinical benefits using a feasible approach. In conjunction with the epidemiological, biochemical and functional data on n-3 fatty acids it seems safe to explore this approach even in primary prevention studies of atherosclerosis.

ACKNOWLEDGMENTS

This work was supported by the Deutsche Forschungsgemeinschaft (project We 681) and the August-Lenz-Stiftung.

REFERENCES

1. Ross R. The pathogenesis of atherosclerosis—an update. *N Engl J Med* 1986;314:488–500.
2. Hamberg M, Svensson J, Samuelsson B. Thromboxanes, a new group of biologically active compounds derived from prostaglandin endoperoxides. *Proc Natl Acad Sci* 1975;72:2994–8.
3. Moncada S, Gryglewski RJ, Bunting S, Vane JR. An enzyme isolated from arteries transforms prostaglandin endoperoxides to an unstable substance that inhibits platelet aggregation. *Nature* 1976;263:663–665.
4. Samuelsson B. Leukotrienes: mediators of immediate hypersensitivity reactions and inflammation. *Science* 1983;220:568–575.
5. Weber, PC. The dietary modification of the arachidonic acid cascade. *Colloque INSERM* 1987;152:119–126.
6. Harker LA. Clinical trials evaluating platelet-modifying drugs in patients with atherosclerotic cardiovascular disease and thrombosis. *Circulation* 1986;73:206–223.
7. Kromann N, Green A. Epidemiological studies in the Upernavik district, Greenland. *Acta Med Scand* 1980;208:401–406.
8. Fischer S, Weber PC, Dyerberg J. The prostacyclin/thromboxane balance is favourably shifted in Greenland Eskimos. *Prostaglandins* 1986;32:235–241.
9. Dyerberg J, Bang HO, Stoffersen E, Moncada S, Vane JR. Eicosapentaenoic acid and prevention of thrombosis and atherosclerosis? *Lancet* 1978;2:117–19.
10. Dyerberg J. Linolenate-derived polyunsaturated fatty acids and prevention of atherosclerosis. *Nutr Rev* 1986;44:125–134.
11. Gordon T. Mortality experience among the Japanese in the United States, Hawaii and California. *Public Health Rep* 1957;72:543–553.
12. Keys A, Kimura N. Diet of middle-aged farmers in Japan. *Am J Clin Nutr* 1970;23:212–223.
13. Yamori Y, Nara Y, Iritani N, Workman RJ, Inagami T. Comparison of serum phospholipid fatty acids among fishing and farming Japanese populations and American inlanders. *J Nutr Sci Vitaminol* (Tokyo) 1985;31:417–422.
14. Goto Y. Serum cholesterol and nutrition in Japan. *Nutr Health* 1985;3:255–257.
15. Weber PC, Fischer S, v. Schacky C, Lorenz R, Strasser T. Dietary omega-3 polyunsaturated fatty acids and eicosanoid formation in man. In: Simopoulos AP, Kifer RR, Martin R, eds. *Health effects of polyunsaturated fatty acids in seafoods.* Orlando: Academic Press. 1986:48–60.
16. Silver MJ, Koch W, Koczis JJ, Ingerman CM, Smith JB. Arachidonic acid causes sudden death in rabbits. *Science* 1974;183:1085–1087.
17. Seyberth HW, Oelz O, Kennedy T, et al. Increased arachidonate in lipids after administration to man: effects on prostaglandin synthesis. *Clin Pharmacol Ther* 1975;18:521–529.

18. Lorenz R, Spengler U, Fischer S, Duhm J, Weber PC. Platelet function, thromboxane formation and blood pressure control during supplementation of the western diet with cod liver oil. *Circulation* 1983;67:504–511.
19. v. Schacky C, Fischer S, Weber PC. Long-term effects of dietary marine n-3 fatty acids upon plasma and cellular lipids, platelet function and eicosanoid formation in humans. *J Clin Invest* 1985;76:1626–1631.
20. Siess W, Roth P, Scherer B, Kurzmann I, Böhlig B, Weber PC. Platelet-membrane fatty acids, platelet aggregation, and thromboxane formation during a mackerel diet. *Lancet* 1980;1:441–444.
21. v. Schacky C, Weber PC. Metabolism and effects on platelet function of the purified eicosapentaenoic and docosahexaenoic acids in humans. *J Clin Invest* 1985;76:2446–2450.
22. Garg M, Wierzbicki A, Thomson A, Clandinin Th. n-3 fatty acids increase the arachidonic acid content of liver cholesterol ester and plasma triacylglyerol fractions in the rat. *Biochem J* 1989;261:11–15.
23. Fischer S, Weber PC. Thromboxane A_3 (TXA3) is formed in human platelets after dietary eicosapentaenoic acid (C20:5n-3). *Biochem Biophys Res Commun* 1983;116:1091–1099.
24. Fischer S, Weber PC. Prostaglandin I_3 is formed in vivo in man after dietary eicosapentaenoic acid. *Nature* (London) 1984;307:165–168.
25. Weber PC, Fischer S, v. Schacky C, Lorenz R, Strasser T. The conversion of dietary eicosapentaenoic acid to prostanoids and leukotrienes in man. *Prog Lipid Res* 1986;25:273–276.
26. Strasser T, Fischer S, Weber PC. Leukotriene B5 is formed in human neutrophils after dietary supplementation with eicosapentaenoic acid. *Proc Natl Acad Sci* 1985;82:1540–1543.
27. Lee TH, Hoover RL, Williams JD, et al. Effect of dietary enrichment with eicosapentaenoic and docosahexaenoic acids in vitro neutrophil and monocyte leukotriene generation and neutrophil function. *N Engl J Med* 1985;312:1217–1224.
28. v. Schacky C, Siess W, Fischer S, Weber PC. A comparative study of eicosapentaenoic acid metabolism by human platelets in vivo and in vitro. *J Lipid Res* 1985;26:457–464.
29. Robinson R, Snyder F. Metabolism of platelet activating factor by rat alveolar macrophages: lyso-PAF as an obligatory intermediate in the formation of alkyl arachidonoyl glycerophospholine species. *Biochem Biophys Acta* 1985;83:52–56.
30. Sugiura T, Masuzawa Y, Waku K. Transacylation of 1-0-alkyl-sn-glycero-3-phosphocholine (lyso platelet activating factor) and 1-0-alkenyl-sn-glycero-3-phosphoethanolamine with docosahexaenoic acid (C22:6n-3). *Biochem Biophys Res Commun* 1985;133:574–580.
31. Daniel LW, Waite M, Wykle RL. A novel mechanism of diglyceride formation. 12-0-tetradecanoylphorbol-13-acetate stimulates the cyclic breakdown and resynthesis of phosphatidylcholine. *J Biol Chem* 1986;261:9128–9131.
32. Fischer S, Vischer A, Preac-Mursic V, Weber PC. Dietary docosahexaenoic acid is retroconverted in man to eicosapentaenoic acid which can be quickly transformed to prostaglandin I3. *Prostaglandins* 1987;34:367–375.
33. Fischer S, v. Schacky C, Siess W, Strasser T, Weber PC. Uptake, release and metabolism of docosahexaenoic acid (DHA, C22:6n-3) in human platelets and neutrophils. *Biochem Biophys Res Commun* 1984;120:907–918.
34. Cooper D, Kelliher G, Kowey P. Modulation of arachidonic acid metabolites and vulnerability to ventricular fibrillation during myocardial ischemia in the cat. *Am Heart J* 1988;116:1194–1200.
35. Sperling R, Robin J-L, Kylander K, Lee T, Lewis R, Austen F. The effects of n-3 polyunsaturated fatty acids on the generation of platelet-activating factor-acether by human monocytes. *J Immunol* 1987;139:4186–4191.
36. Landymore RW, MacAulay M, Sheridan B, Cameron C. Comparison of cod liver oil and aspirin-dipyridamole for the prevention of intimal hyperplasia in autologous vein grafts. *Ann Thorac Surg* 1986;41:54–57.
37. Weiner BH, Ockene IS, Levine PH, et al. Inhibition of atherosclerosis by cod liver oil in a hyperlipidemic swine model. *N Engl J Med* 1986;315:841–846.
38. Davis HR, Bridenstine RT, Vesselinovitch D, Wissler RW. Fish oil inhibits development of atherosclerosis in rhesus monkeys. *Arteriosclerosis* 1987;7:441–449.
39. Barcelli U, Glas-Greenwalt P, Pollak V. Enhancing effect of dietary supplementation with n-3 fatty acids on plasma fibrinolysis in normal subjects. *Thromb Res* 1985;39:307–312.

40. Endres S, Ghorbani R, Kelley V, et al. The effect of dietary supplementation with n-3 polyunsaturated fatty acids on the synthesis of inter-leukin-1 and tumor necrosis factor by mononuclear cells. *N Engl J Med* 1989;320:265–271.
41. Fox P, DiCorleto P. Fish oils inhibit endothelial cell production of platelet-derived growth factor-like protein. *Science* 1988;241:453–456.
42. Shimokawa H, Lam J, Chesebro J, Bowie E, Vanhoutte P. Effects of dietary supplementation with cod-liver oil on endothelium-dependent responses in porcine coronary arteries. *Circulation* 1987;76:898–905.
43. Cartwright IJ, Pockley AG, Jalloway JH, Greaves M, Preston FE. The effect of dietary n-3 polyunsaturated fatty acids on erythrocyte deformability and blood viscosity in healthy volunteers *Atherosclerosis* 1985;55:267–281.
44. Wahlquist M, Lo C, Myers K. Fish intake and arterial wall characteristics in healthy people and diabetic patients. *Lancet* 1989;2:944–946.
45. Eaton S, Konner M. Paleolithic nutrition. A consideration of its nature and current implications. *N Engl J Med* 1985;312:283–289.
46. Grigg LE, Kay T, Valentine PA. Determinantes of restenosis and lack of effect of dietary supplementation with eicosapentaenoic acid on the incidence of coronary artery restenosis after angioplasty. *J Am Coll Cardiol* 1989;13:665–672.
47. Dehmer GJ, Popma JJ, van der Berg EK, et al. Reduction in the rate of early restenosis after coronary angioplasty by a diet supplemented with n-3 fatty acids. *N Engl J Med* 1988;319:733–740.
48. Slack JD, Pinkerton CA, van Tassel J, et al. Can oral fish oil supplement minimize restenoisis after percutaneous translumenal coronary angioplasty? [Abstract.] *J Am Coll Cardiol* 1987;9:64a.
49. Milner M, Gallino R, Leffingwell A, Pichard A, Rosenberg J, Lindsay J. High dose omega-3 fatty acid supplementation reduces clinical restenosis after coronary angioplasty. *Circulation* 1988;78 (suppl II) 634.
50. Reis G, Boucher Th, Sipperly M, et al. Randomised trial of fish oil for prevention of restenosis after coronary angioplasty. *Lancet* 1989;2:177–181.
51. Kromhout D, Bosschieter EB, Coulander CDL. The inverse relation between fish consumption and 20-year mortality from coronary heart disease. *N Engl J Med* 1985;312:1205–1209.
52. Norell SE, Ahlbom A, Feychting M, Pedersen NL. Fish consumption and mortality from coronary heart disease. *Br Med J* 1986;293:426.
53. Shekelle RB, Missel L, Oglesby P, Shryock AM, Stamler, J. Fish consumption and mortality from coronary heart disease (letter). *N Engl J Med* 1985;313:820.
54. Burr M, Fehily A, Gilbert J, et al. Effects of changes in fat, fish and fibre intakes on death and myocardial reinfarction: diet and reinfarction trial (DART). *Lancet* 1989;2:757–761.
55. Weber PC. Ist man, was man isst? Nahrungs-und Membran-fettsauren, Zellfunktionen und Zivilisationskraukheiten. 114 Vers. GDNÄ, Wissenschaffliche Verlagsgesell Schaft mbH, Stuttgart, 1986:187–194.

Atherosclerosis Reviews, Volume 21,
edited by A. Leaf and P. C. Weber.
Raven Press, Ltd., New York © 1990.

The Oslo Study:

Some Trial Results

Ingvar Hjermann

*Department of Medicine, Medical Out-Patient Clinic, Oslo University Medical School,
Ullevaal Hospital, 0407 Oslo 4, Norway*

The Oslo Study of cardiovascular diseases includes epidemiological studies and preventive trials. One of these trials was the primary preventive randomized trial on the effect of diet and smoking intervention on the incidence of coronary heart disease (CHD) (1,2). In this paper I will present the main 5-year and $8\frac{1}{2}$-year results, and discuss why the intervention strategy in this trial seemed to be more effective than it was in other trials, including the drug trials with end points of clinical events and total mortality.

This 5-year trial (observation time: 5 to $6\frac{1}{2}$ years) included 1,232 healthy men, aged 40 to 49 years, at relatively high risk of CHD, i.e., with serum cholesterol in the range 6.9 to 9.0 mmol/L, with an average 7.6 mmol/L at baseline. Eighty percent of the men were daily cigarette smokers and all participants had a systolic blood pressure of <150 mm Hg at the last (third) examination before randomization.

The men in the intervention group were recommended to lower their blood lipids by change of diet and to stop smoking. The main diet strategy was a substantial reduction in saturated fat with a relatively small increase in polyunsaturates. In addition, a reduced body weight in all overweight men was attempted.

Mean serum cholesterol was lowered by 13% in the intervention group (from an average of three measurements before randomization to an average of yearly measured values during the trial). The net difference in cholesterol levels between the two groups during the 5 years of the trial was 10%. Mean fasting and nonfasting triglycerides fell by approximately 20% to 30%, respectively. Twenty-five percent of the smokers stopped smoking compared to 17% in the control group who stopped (Fig. 1).

Diagnosis of events during the trial was made blindly according to predefined criteria, by cardiologists not involved in the study. Main end points were myocardial infarction (MI) (fatal and nonfatal) and sudden death (SD). At the end of the observation period, the incidence of MI and SD was 47% lower in the

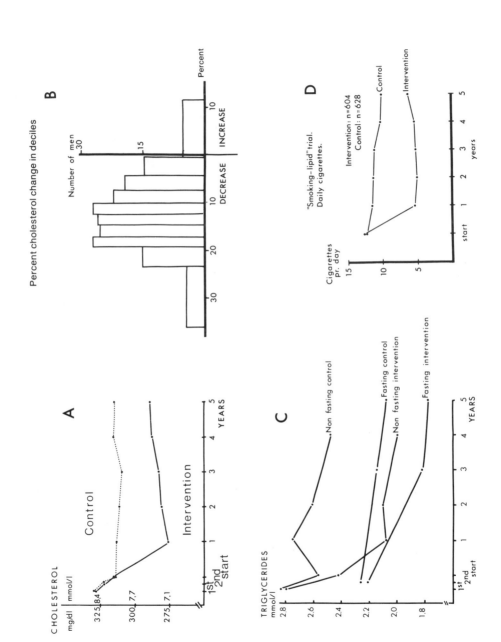

Percent cholesterol change in deciles

TABLE 1. *Oslo study: diet–antismoking trial—cardiovascular events*

	Intervention (*n* = 604)		Control (*n* = 628)	
	No. of events	Rates (0/00)	No. of events	Rates (0/00)
Sudden coronary deaths	3	5	11	18
Sudden unexplained death	0	—	1	2
Sudden coronary + unexplained death	3	5	12	19[a]
Fatal MI	3	5	2	3
Fatal MI + sudden death	6	10	14	22[b]
Nonfatal MI	13	22	22	35[c]
Total coronary events	19	31	36	57[d]
Fatal stroke	2	3	1	2
Nonfatal stroke	1	2	2	3
Total cardiovascular events	22	36	39	62[e]
Bypass surgery	1	2	3	5

Note: two-sided tests.
One event: the "hardest" counted in each person, see text.
[a] $p = 0.024$.
[b] $p = 0.086$.
[c] $p = 0.153$.
[d] $p = 0.028$.
[e] $p - 0.038$.

intervention group than in the controls ($p = 0.028$, two-tailed log rank test). When the incidence of stroke was added the difference was still significant (Table 1).

This study, with only 1,232 healthy men, was not expected to show a difference in mortality because of the relatively few expected mortality events during the observation time. However, total mortality turned out to be 33% lower in the intervention group (16 vs. 24), although statistically significant only for the subgroup of sudden coronary death.

Therefore, the conclusion of the 5-year trial was that advice to change eating habits and to stop smoking significantly reduced the incidence of first MI and SD. Statistical analysis by the Cox's proportional hazards model indicated that the reduction in incidence in the intervention group correlated significantly with the reduction in total cholesterol and nonsignificantly with the reduction in smoking.

$8\frac{1}{2}$-YEAR RESULTS

During the trial, the men in the intervention group met for examination and counseling every sixth month (the control group met every twelfth month). Af-

FIG. 1. Oslo Study: (**A, B**) intervention effects on serum cholesterol, (**C**) triglycerides, and (**D**) smoking. Pipe smoking is included; 50 g pipe tobacco/week equals 7 cigarettes/day.

ter the end of the trial, the participants were not called for until another $3\frac{1}{2}$ years had elapsed. At this point, we did not expect to find the mean serum cholesterol at the same low level as at the end of the trial, as no counseling had taken place during the $3\frac{1}{2}$ years. However, we found that mean total cholesterol had not changed during these $3\frac{1}{2}$ years in the intervention group, whereas it had been reduced in the controls, probably due to the fact that all participants had been informed about the 5-year results.

The differences between the groups in the incidence of coronary heart disease and mortality were maintained after 102 months (Fig. 2 and Table 2). This finding is of particular interest, as the risk-factor differences between the groups diminished after the end of the trial. It seems, therefore, that the preventive effect of the earlier and greater differences in risk-factor levels was still present. However, when comparing the number of total coronary events that occurred at the end of the trial (19 in the intervention group and 36 in the control group) with the number that occurred in the 102-month follow-up (25 in the intervention group and 45 in the control group), there is a difference of six in the intervention group and of nine in the control group, pointing to a decreasing difference in the coronary heart disease rate. This finding is in concordance with the decreasing net difference in risk factors.

The study was not designed to reveal significant differences in total mortality between the groups. Therefore, it should be noted that after 102 months, the

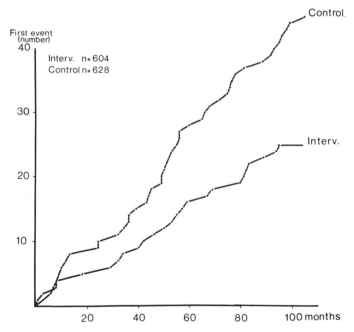

FIG. 2. Oslo Study—diet–smoking trial: cumulative incidence of coronary events (i.e., fatal and nonfatal myocardial infarction and sudden death) at the 102-month follow-up shows the same trend as at 60 months. Three participants were lost to follow-up but were alive.

TABLE 2. *Oslo study. Diet–antismoking trial*[a]

	Intervention ($n = 604$)	Control ($n = 628$)
Sudden coronary death	4	12
Sudden unexplained death	0	1
MI	3	4
Stroke	2	1
Cancer	6	10
Suicide/violent	4	2
Pneumonia	0	1
Total mortality	19	31

[a] $8\frac{1}{2}$-year results, mortality events.
$p = 0.055$ (one-tail test).

difference in total mortality has increased from 33% to 40%, and the difference became marginally significant, with $p = 0.055$ (not accounting for multiple testing). The use of a one-sided test is controversial. It might be argued that a two-sided test should be used always in controlled trials, because the results could be expected to go in either direction. The question is whether there is any reason to expect the results in this nondrug trial to favor the control group.

Independent of one-sided or two-sided tests, the results show significant differences for sudden death, sudden coronary death, and total coronary events. Even bypass surgery (originally not defined as an end point) seems to be significantly more frequent in the control group. Thus, the results for the incidence of coronary surgery are in the same direction as are the main incidence and mortality figures, which strengthen the results as a whole.

The Strategy of Prevention

Two other trials in primary prevention of CHD have been reported relatively recently: the Lipid Research Clinic (LRC) trial with cholestyramine (3) and the Helsinki Heart trial with gemfibrozil (4). Both trials showed significant effects on CHD incidence, although it displayed less of an effect than it did in the Oslo Study. In addition, the results of the Oslo trial consistently showed results in the same direction for all main coronary end points, as well as for bypass surgery and total mortality. The great problem for drug trials in prevention of CHD has been the lack of effect on total mortality, except possibly for trials with nicotinic acid.

If our nondrug approach is more effective, what could be the reason? Apart from the effect of cholesterol lowering and the possible effect of the relatively small net difference in smoking between the groups, nonfasting triglycerides were reduced by almost 30% in the intervention group, and body weight was reduced almost 3 kg on the average. Qualitatively, the lipid-lowering diet mainly aimed at a reduction of saturated fatty acids and an increase in complex carbohydrates, fiber, and fish products. Such a diet also reduces blood pressure, increases glucose tolerance, and reduces the frequently increased postprandial insulin in these hyperlipidemic men. We have shown also that such a dietary regimen normalizes a more or less defective fibrinolytic capacity and the elevated coagulation factor VII, frequently seen in sedentary men with elevated lipids, especially triglycerides. We have shown also that in this population, elevated blood lipids and mild hypertension very often appear together in the same individual, and that in such individuals there is a positive correlation between arterial catecholamines and blood cholesterol.

Probably a great proportion of coronary high-risk men have disturbances in two or more of the factors named above. It seems from our studies that most of these factors are influenced in the potential beneficial direction by the change in eating habits. If this is not the case for the drug trials (and this is certainly *not* so for the antihypertensive trials with diuretics and β-blockers), one might speculate whether such metabolic effects could be one reason for the apparently greater effect on CHD of our nondrug intervention.

NONPHARMACOLOGICAL TREATMENT OF BLOOD PRESSURE

In a recent trial we have shown also that if we add salt and alcohol reduction to this lipid- and body-weight-reducing regimen, mild hypertension (diastolic 94 to 104 mm Hg) can be treated successfully in an intervention group compared to controls in a randomized trial, (net difference in mean blood pressure between the groups after 1 year: 9 mm for standing and 8 mm for supine blood pressure). However, in such a trial, the blood pressure difference could well be of lesser importance than could be the effects of both the "metabolic" variables cited above (i.e., blood lipids, glucose tolerance, blood insuline, catecholamines) and the hemostatic risk factors (i.e., impaired fibrinolytic capacity, elevated coagulation factor VII, and increased platelet activity).

An important field of research in the years to come will be the search for antihypertensive drugs that not only lower blood pressure but also change all these "metabolic" variables in the supposed beneficial direction.

REFERENCES

1. Hjermann I, Byre KV, Holme I, Leren P. Effect of diet and smoking intervention on the incidence of coronary heart disease. Report from the Oslo Study Group of a randomized trial in healthy men. *Lancet* 1981;2:1303–1310.
2. Hjermann I, Holme I, Leren P. Oslo Study diet and antismoking trial. Results after 102 months. *Am J Med* 1986;80(Suppl 2 A):7–11.
3. Lipid Research Clinics Program. The Lipid Research Clinics Coronary Primary Prevention Trial results. I. Reduction in incidence of coronary heart disease. *JAMA* 1984;251:351–364.
4. Frick MH, Elo O, Haapa K, et al. Helsinki Heart Study: Primary-prevention trial with gemfibrozil in middle-aged men with dyslipidemia. Safety of treatment, changes in risk factors, and incidence of coronary heart disease. *N Engl J Med* 1987;317:1237–1245.

Atherosclerosis Reviews, Volume 21,
edited by A. Leaf and P. C. Weber.
Raven Press, Ltd., New York © 1990.

The North Karelia Project:

Results of a Major National Demonstration Project on CHD Prevention in Finland Since 1972

Pekka Puska, Erkki Vartiainen, Heikki J. Korhonen,
Leena Kartovaara, Mari-Anna Berg, Pirjo Pietinen,
Aulikki Nissinen, and Jaakko Tuomilehto

*Department of Epidemiology, National Public Health Institute,
SF-00300 Helsinki, Finland*

The great burden of cardiovascular diseases (CVD), and especially that of coronary heart disease (CHD), became obvious by the beginning of the 1970s in most industrialized countries, and particularly so in Finland. Previous research had identified not only the extent of the problem and geographical differences in disease rates, but also certain factors consistently and independently associated with the risk of CHD. Following the results of many descriptive prospective epidemiological studies several intervention trials were proposed and launched.

Mortality statistics already showed in the 1960s that Finland had the highest CHD mortality rates, especially among men. These differences were confirmed by a World Health Organization (WHO) myocardial infarction study (1) and by the Seven Countries Study (2). This information added to the public concern, especially in the province of North Karelia, which had the highest rates in Finland (3). In January 1971 the representatives of North Karelia signed a petition in which they asked the national government to "take urgent action to reduce the high CVD rates in the area."

After the petition planning started, it involved local authorities, Finnish experts, and the World Health Organization. The available medical and epidemiological information was viewed. Attention was drawn to the likely causal roles of certain risk factors, especially raised serum [low-density lipoprotein (LDL)] cholesterol, high blood pressure, and smoking. Information was available about the very high occurrence of these risk factors among the North Karelian male population. Particularly high international comparisons were made with the average serum cholesterol level, obviously largely due to the high consumption of dairy fat.

In the planning phase attention was drawn to the obvious problems of classical randomized trials "to give the final proof" on the causality of the risk factors. Many pointed out that the mass epidemic of CHD is due to the generally high levels of the risk factors, related to the general lifestyles and their social and cultural determinants. Would it not be more logical and effective to change the community instead of some of its individuals only?

The initial situation in North Karelia, together with these considerations, led to the adoption of a community-based approach in the North Karelia Project, thus becoming the first major community-based study on the prevention of CHD. The decision was supported further by the fact that the cessation of smoking, certain dietary modifications, and the control of high blood pressure should be useful, safe, and promote health, in general.

THE IMPLEMENTATION OF THE PROJECT

The intervention was started in North Karelia in 1972 after completion of the large baseline survey. The baseline survey as well as several other information sources were used to make a community diagnosis—i.e., to understand the various determinants and change the possibilities of the target risk factors. The general aim was to reduce the high occurrence of the target risk factors and to promote general risk-reducing lifestyle changes in the whole population. The method was a comprehensive and innovative intervention through the various community organizations and together with the community, emphasizing the involvement of the population itself.

The idea was to carry out a systematic and comprehensive intervention using the epidemiological knowledge of the risk factors on one side and relevant behavioral and social sciences principles on the other. The target risk factors were chosen using available epidemiological knowledge about their role and information on their occurrence in the local population. The practical intervention activities were integrated in the existing service structure and social organization of the area. The role of the project has been to define the objectives, and to train, coordinate, and promote the activities, as well as to assess the results, with most of the actual work being done by the community itself.

The comprehensive educational and service-oriented program to modify the risk factor profile of the population on North Karelia was based on local community action and a local service structure. A central aim was to promote lifestyles that reduced the risk factor levels and promote health. Practical skills were taught, social support for change was provided, and environmental modifications were arranged as part of the comprehensive community organization for change.

The large baseline survey of the North Karelia Project was carried out in the spring of 1972 in North Karelia and in the chosen reference area. Thereafter, the special intervention was started in North Karelia. After the initial 5 years (since 1977), the project (as a national demonstration program) actively became involved in national efforts to reduce activities that were known risks, thus also influencing the population in the control area.

After 10 years the program was enlarged to include a more integrated prevention of major noncommunicable diseases (NCD) and promotion of health. This was associated with the respective WHO programs ("CINDI" and "INTER-HEALTH"). Simultaneously, major activities were launched to prevent risk factors developing in young people. Meanwhile, the national involvement continued. After the 15-year survey was completed a decision was made to intensify CHD prevention, focusing particularly on action to reduce cholesterol levels and the incidence of smoking.

EVALUATION OF THE PROJECT

The major questions of the project evaluation were whether it was possible to influence the risk factor levels in the population and, if so, whether such changes led to changes in CHD rates. For this evaluation a quasi-experimental study design was formulated. Changes in the North Karelian population were compared with changes in another reference area with similar characteristics to those of North Karelia.

The assessment of the effect of the intervention of health behavior and risk factors was based on repeated independent surveys of large representative population samples (30 to 59 years) in North Karelia and in a matched reference area at the outset (spring 1972), and after successive 5-year periods (1977, 1982, and 1987). In the initial assessments, the net reduction in North Karelia (the reduction in North Karelia minus the reduction in the reference area) was judged to have been as a result of the program. This estimate was conservative because the project probably influences developments not only in the reference area but nationally as well.

Because of the national activities of the project since 1977, the original reference area could no more be considered as a "control area." However, the developments in North Karelia were compared subsequently with those in the rest of Finland. In the 1982 and in later surveys a third survey area in South West Finland was used and the surveys have been implemented as part of the MON-ICA project.

Independent random samples have been used in the surveys to assess the magnitude of changes in the whole population. Special follow-up studies of cohorts have been done additionally to analyze the changes among individuals. Strictly standardized and similar questionnaires and methods have been used on large samples in the survey areas.

Since 1978 annual surveys have been carried out by mail for independent representative samples of the population (15 to 64 years) in both all of Finland and in North Karelia only. The aim of these surveys has been to monitor more rapidly the health behavior changes and to serve the process evaluation.

TABLE 1. *Sample size (n) and participation rates (%) in population surveys*
(30 to 59-year-old population)

| | North Karelia | | | | Kuopio County | | | |
| | Men | | Women | | Men | | Women | |
Year	n	%	n	%	n	%	n	%
1972	1959	94	2056	96	2918	91	2949	94
1977	2063	87	2020	91	2933	89	2996	92
1982	1599	77	1511	84	1459	83	1143	88
1987	1521	79	1485	87	762	82	744	87

The disease rates in North Karelia have been monitored by special myocardial infarction and stroke registers that operate in the whole of North Karelia using WHO criteria. The mortality trends have been analyzed based on national mortality data since 1969, the year when ICD-8 classification was adopted and which has been used in Finland throughout the period presented here. Thus, three preprogram years are included. Age-adjusted rates for men aged 35 to 64 years have been used.

In addition to the effect evaluation, the overall evaluation of the project has been concerned with the assessment of the feasibility of the preventive activities of various process factors in the community, of the costs involved, and of the broader overall consequences of the activity. The evaluation methods and the evaluation results have been published in numerous other publications (4–7).

RESULTS OF THE PROJECT

The sample sizes and the participation rates in the four main surveys are shown in Table 1. Table 2 gives a summary of the 15-year results on risk factors.

TABLE 2. *Level of risk factors in North Karelia, Kuopio County, and South-West Finland from 1972 to 1987 in population surveys (30 to 59-year-old population)*

| | Percent of current smokers | | Serum cholesterol (mmol/L) | | Diastolic blood pressure (mm Hg) | |
	North Karelia	Kuopio County	North Karelia	Kuopio County	North Karelia	Kuopio County
Men						
1972	52	50	7.09	6.85	92.0	93.3
1977	44	45	6.68	6.74	88.6	92.6
1982	36	42	6.25	6.20	88.1	89.1
1987	36	41	6.25	6.20	88.1	89.1
Women						
1972	10	11	6.98	6.82	92.4	91.3
1977	10	12	6.56	6.48	86.3	88.4
1982	15	15	6.11	6.01	84.5	84.8
1987	16	15	5.98	5.86	83.2	83.9

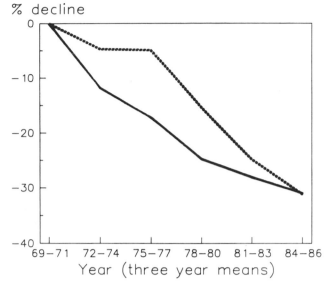

FIG. 1. Percentage decline in CHD mortality of 35- to 64-year-old men in North Karelia (NK; —) and in the rest of Finland (SF; ---).

The results of Table 2 show major changes in North Karelia during the first 10 years, and substantial although statistically significant smaller changes in the reference area (for men $p < 0.01$ for all the risk factors). Thereafter, the changes in North Karelia and in the two other areas have been small. Among men, the smoking rates in North Karelia in 1987 were lower than they were elsewhere; the serum cholesterol and blood pressure levels were still high and higher still than they were in South-West Finland.

Figure 1 shows the decline in age-adjusted CHD mortality rates among men in North Karelia and in the rest of Finland after the three preprogram years and

TABLE 3. Regression-based change in CHD mortality between 1969 to 1987 men, age 35 to 64 years

	North Karelia		Rest of Finland	
	Men	Women	Men	Women
Annual decline				
1969 to 1977	18.2%	7.2%	3.0%	2.6%
p value	0.005	0.0009	0.144	0.0006
1978 to 1987	9.6%	0.7%	15.3%	2.1%
p value	0.016	0.670	0.0001	0.0014
Interactions				
Area-year	NS	NS		
Area-period	0.006	0.034		
Area-period-year	0.001	0.003		

TABLE 4. *Regression-based annual decline in age-adjusted mortality of total cancer among people 30 to 64 years old*

Period	North Karelia	Reference area	Rest of Finland
1969 to 1973	−6.3	−6.6	−3.2
1974 to 1978	−4.5	+3.2[a]	−1.9
1979 to 1983	−13.9	+0.6	−5.7[b]

[a,b] Statistical significance of difference in relation to North Karelia.

is based on the means of three consecutive years. The decline in North Karelia was steep in the 1970s but slowed down in the 1980s. Toward the middle of the 1980s, the decline throughout Finland reached that of North Karelia. Between 1974 to 1979 North Karelia had the largest difference in decline compared with the rest of Finland or with the reference area (8).

Table 3 shows the regression-based decline in CHD mortality (age group: 35 to 64 years) for 1969 to 1977 and 1978 to 1987, respectively. During the first period, the decline in North Karelia was 18% among men while in the rest of the country it was only 3% ($p < 0.001$). During the second period, the declines were 10% and 15%, respectively.

Table 4 shows the annual mean decline in age-adjusted mortality of total cancer incidence for three 5-year periods. The results show that—unlike

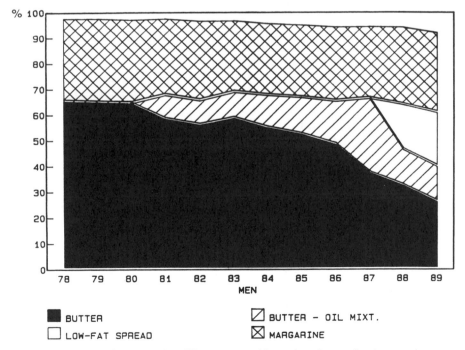

FIG. 2. Percentage of people using different types of fat on bread according to annual surveys in 1978 to 1989 among men aged 15 to 64 years across Finland.

CHD—a major reduction and difference in reduction in favor of NK did not occur between 1974 and 1978 but later on, from 1979 to 1983.

Other evaluation results have demonstrated the rather even distribution of the risk factor changes in the various groups of the population, as well a net reduction in the CVD-related disability rates (4). An improvement in the subjective health of the North Karelia population was observed as a consequence of the program (6).

The annual health behavior monitoring surveys show some major dietary changes in association with the new cholesterol reduction activities since 1987 nationally and in North Karelia. Figure 2 shows the trend in the choice of fat spread, a major source of fat intake in Finland. Particularly after 1987, as a result of educational efforts and legislative changes, the consumption of butter is diminishing rapidly while that of vegetable oil–based products is increasing.

DISCUSSION AND CONCLUSIONS

The North Karelia Project became the first major community-based demonstration project in the field of CVD largely because of the historical reasons mentioned previously: high disease rates, high general risk factor levels, and the petition from the local people. At the same time, we must acknowledge the importance of the previous research work in Finland, of the international collaboration revealing the major risk factors, and of the support from WHO and other agencies to launch the program in North Karelia.

The implementation of the program has been good throughout the 15-year period. Local health services and their staff have cooperated well, thus forming the backbone for the activities. The local population has participated readily in the activities, and various community organizations have contributed in various ways to the aims of the project in the area. Because the project aims were integrated within the existing health services and because broad community participation was a key feature, the overall costs of the program have been modest.

To influence people's health-related lifestyles is not easy. Even when the hazards of unhealthy habits are well known, many intervention activities meet with limited or no success. The results and experiences presented here indicate major changes and show that, at least in favorable conditions, comprehensive, determined and well-planned community-based action can lead to substantial favorable changes.

It is hard to pinpoint the reason for this favorable effect in North Karelia and whether and how it could be accomplished elsewhere. A community program like this ultimately tests whether a specific program as a whole (which should be designated so that it can be applied on a larger scale) is feasible and effective under given conditions. The impact of various community conditions and of different components of the project on successes and failures can be evaluated only to a limited extent.

Major obstacles to the project, particularly at the start, were shortages of health service resources, many socioeconomic problems and the linkage of high-fat intake with local dairy farming and with long-standing cultural habits. Strong favourable factors were the people's awareness of the problem and their motivation to do something, systematic service structure, a good data base, and support from national and local administrations. The project team feels that, in addition, attention to relevant behavioral and social theories and a lot of practical dedicated, hard work in the field have contributed to success.

In spite of the substantial reduction in the risk factor levels and CHD rates, the mortality of CHD in North Karelia and in all of Finland is still high by international standards. This, together with the leveling off of the risk factor trends, led to the launching of a new intensified intervention after 1987 in North Karelia. These activities are linked closely with recent national initiatives where the Project is involved also. Because the most outstanding risk factor today seems to be the still very high serum cholesterol level, the major emphasis in the program is on general cholesterol-reducing dietary changes. The interim monitoring shows, indeed, remarkable recent changes in the target nutritional habits. However, only the 20-year follow-up population survey in 1992 and a respective mortality follow-up will show the possible effects of these efforts on desired risk factor reductions, on CHD mortality changes, and on the overall health of the population.

In conclusion, the experiences and results show that well-conceived, comprehensive, community-based programs can have a positive effect on lifestyles and on cardiovascular risk factors for a whole population and that such a development is associated with reduced cardiovascular mortality rates. Furthermore, they demonstrate the potential of a community-based approach in changing the risk factors as well as giving practical experience in organizing such activities within health services and other community settings. The national experiences show that a major practical demonstration project can be a powerful tool for promoting favorable national developments.

REFERENCES

1. WHO. Myocardial infarction community registers. Public Health in Europe No. 5. Regional Office for Europe. Copenhagen: World Health Organization, 1976.
2. Keys A. *Seven Countries. A multivariate analysis of death and coronary heart disease.* Cambridge: Harvard University Press, MA, 1980:381.
3. Pohjola S, Siltanen P, Romo M, et al. Sydäninfarktin esiintyvyys ja ennuste Suomessa vuonna 1973. Helsingin, Turun, Tampereen ja Pohjois-Karjalan rekistereiden vertailua. *Duodecim* 1980;96:18–23.
4. Puska P, Tuomilehto J, Salonen J, et al. Community control of cardiovascular diseases—the North Karelia project: Evaluation of a comprehensive community programme for control of cardiovascular diseases in 1972–77 in North Karelia. Copenhagen: WHO/EURO, 1981:Monograph series.
5. Puska P, Salonen J, Nissinen A, et al. Change in risk factors for coronary heart disease during 10 years of a community intervention programme (North Karelia project). *Br Med J* 1983;287: 1840–1844.

6. Puska P, Nissinen A, Salonen JT, et al. The community-based strategy to prevent coronary heart disease: conclusions from the ten years of the North Karelia project. *Annu Rev Public Health* 1985;6:147–193.
7. Tuomilehto J, Geboers J, Salonen J, Nissinen A, Kuulasmaa K, Puska P. Decline in cardiovascular mortality in North Karelia and other parts of Finland. *Br Med J* 1986;293:1068–1071.
8. Salonen JT, Puska P, Kottke TE, Tuomilehto J, Nissinen A. Decline in mortality from coronary heart disease in Finland from 1969 to 1979. *Br Med J* 1983;286:1857–1860.

Atherosclerosis Reviews, Volume 21,
edited by A. Leaf and P. C. Weber.
Raven Press, Ltd., New York © 1990.

Relationship of Triglyceride and High-Density Lipoprotein Metabolism

Gero Miesenböck and Josef R. Patsch

Division of Clinical Atherosclerosis Research, Department of Medicine,
University of Innsbruck, A-6020 Innsbruck, Austria

Low plasma levels of high-density lipoproteins (HDL) predict an increased risk for coronary artery disease (CAD) at the population level (1,2). Since the negative association between HDL–cholesterol and CAD is at least as strong as that of all other known risk factors (3), it is tempting to attribute to HDL a causally protective role against atherosclerosis and to assign to elevating HDL–cholesterol levels part of the CAD risk reduction reported in intervention trials (4). The biochemical framework of this "causalist" school of thinking is the reverse cholesterol transport hypothesis (5): According to this hypothesis, cholesterol from cellular membranes is trapped in HDL by esterification with phosphatidylcholine-derived fatty acids. This reaction is catalyzed by the HDL-associated enzyme lecithin:cholesterol acyltransferase (LCAT) (5). Esterification blocks the hydroxyl group of cholesterol and thus prevents the rediffusion of cholesterol to the cell membrane. A lipid transfer protein (LTP-I) present in plasma eventually transfers the cholesteryl esters from HDL to lipoproteins of lower density (6,7) which are removed via specific receptors by the liver (8,9). Alternatively, cholesterol-laden HDL might themselves acquire apolipoprotein (apo) E, a ligand that allows their direct removal by hepatic receptors (10). In this way, cholesterol is returned from peripheral cells to the liver for excretion into the bile.

Considering the epidemiologic data, the causalist view delineated above would imply that reverse cholesterol transport is impaired at low HDL levels. In turn, interventions raising HDL–cholesterol would reestablish the proper function of the reverse cholesterol transport system. Evidence in support of this notion, however, is lacking.

An alternative view regarding the negative association of HDL–cholesterol with CAD is based on the intimate relationship that exists between the metabolism of triglyceride-rich (TG-rich) lipoproteins and that of HDL and its major subfractions: One of them, HDL_3, consists of small, lipid-poor and dense particles. The other fraction, HDL_2, comprises larger, more lipid-rich and less dense particles (11–13). Of the two HDL subfractions, HDL_3 is present in the plasma at rather constant concentration, but HDL_2 levels vary greatly and thus account for most of the variability of total HDL–cholesterol (14,15). Hence, the negative association of HDL–cholesterol and CAD risk is essentially due to the variable plasma levels of HDL_2 (16,17). By the same token, the relationship between triglycerides and HDL is—at a close look—one between triglycerides and HDL_2.

EVIDENCE FOR THE TRIGLYCERIDE–HDL_2 CONNECTION

1.   In the postabsorptive state, the plasma levels of TG-rich lipoproteins and HDL_2 are inversely related (18–20). The association becomes much stronger in the postprandial state (20).

2.   This latter correlation does not only hold in cross-sectional studies but also in the longitudinal follow-up of individuals where drastic interventions changed triglyceride concentrations in the postprandial state and HDL_2 levels reciprocally. When aerobic exercise such as running raised HDL_2, postprandial lipemia was attenuated, and when injury forced cessation of exercise, both HDL_2 concentration and postprandial lipemia returned—reciprocally—to their basal values recorded at the beginning of the trial (20).

3.   The activities of the two major triglyceride-metabolizing enzymes in the circulation, i.e., lipoprotein lipase and hepatic lipase (21–23), are correlated to the plasma levels of HDL_2. Hepatic lipase activity is inversely related to HDL_2 (15,24). Under certain conditions (see below), HDL_2 serves as a substrate for this enzyme. In contrast, lipoprotein lipase varies positively with HDL_2 (15,25). However, lipoprotein lipase does not act on HDL but hydrolyzes large TG-rich lipoproteins. Hence, HDL_2 must be affected by this process indirectly.

4.   Drugs that raise HDL concentrations lower TG-rich lipoproteins in at least one of two ways (26): They either decrease the synthesis of TG-rich lipoproteins (nicotinic acid, fibric acid derivatives) or accelerate their catabolism by lipoprotein lipase (fibric acid derivatives). A mechanism by which these drugs would raise HDL levels directly is not known.

TRIGLYCERIDES AND HDL: FROM CORRELATIONS TO CAUSE AND EFFECT

The close correlation between TG-rich lipoproteins and HDL suggests a causal relationship between the two lipoprotein families. We now provide evidence that it is the metabolism of TG-rich lipoproteins that affects HDL and not vice versa. TG-rich lipoproteins exert their influence on HDL levels both via catabolism and formation of the susceptible fraction HDL_2.

Triglycerides and the Catabolism of HDL_2

The catabolism of HDL_2 to smaller HDL_3 requires the action of hepatic lipase. This is dramatically illustrated by hepatic lipase deficiency (27,28): In this familial condition, HDL_2 is the dominant HDL species in plasma, and HDL_3 is virtually absent. For HDL_2 to become an appropriate substrate for hepatic lipase, its composition has to be changed from a cholesteryl ester-rich into a cholesteryl ester-deficient, triglyceride-enriched particle.

This compositional requirement for catabolism of HDL_2 was demonstrated in normotriglycerdemic subjects during the course of postprandial lipemia (29), where the concentration of TG-rich lipoproteins changes most under physiologic circumstances. In going from the postabsorptive (pa) state to the postprandial (pp) state, HDL_2 showed moderate enrichment with phospholipids, which was independent of the magnitude of postprandial lipemia. There was also enrichment of the HDL_2 particles with triglycerides. However, this enrichment depended on the magnitude of postprandial lipemia: In individuals with low-level lipemia, there was little if any postprandial enrichment with triglycerides, while in individuals with high-level lipemia, HDL_2 became considerably enriched with triglycerides (29). These compositional changes indicate that clearance of TG-rich lipoproteins in the circulation—at any rate—provides excess phospholipids that associate with pa HDL_2 to form phospholipid-enriched pp HDL_2. The rate of clearance, however, determines to what extent cholesteryl esters in pa HDL_2 will be replaced by triglycerides in pp HDL_2. If this occurs in a high enough proportion, the threshold for conversion of an HDL_2 into an HDL_3 particle has been crossed:

Hepatic lipase removes excess phospholipids from HDL_2; if the enzyme is immunologically blocked *in vivo,* phospholipids accumulate in HDL (30,31). Apart from this phospholipase A_1 activity, hepatic lipase is a triacylglycerol hydrolase (21–23). Therefore, the enzyme will catabolize both phospholipids and triglycerides of pp HDL_2 down to the limit set by the nondegradable cholesteryl esters remaining in the HDL_2 core (29): When triglyceride-poor, cholesteryl ester-rich pp HDL_2 from individuals with low postprandial lipemia are subjected to hepatic lipase action, there is not enough hydrolyzable triglyceride substrate in the core of HDL_2 to reduce its size to HDL_3; hence, the product particle will be a relatively phospholipid-depleted HDL_2. On the contrary, triglyceride-rich, cholesteryl ester-deficient pp HDL_2 from individuals with high postprandial lipemia provide sufficient triglyceride substrate in their core to be converted into smaller HDL_3 (Fig. 1).

Fulfillment of the compositional requirement for HDL_2 catabolism is made possible by LTP-I, which catalyzes the heteroexchange of triglycerides and cholesteryl esters between TG-rich lipoproteins and HDL (6,7). An inherited deficiency of LTP-I due to a gene-splicing defect has been described in two siblings (32). In this condition, the transfer of nondiffusible core lipids between lipoproteins is impossible. One would expect that even repetitive cycles of high postprandial lipemia would be unable to direct triglycerides into HDL_2, thus preventing their catabolism. Indeed, the two LTP-I-deficient patients exhibited extremely high HDL–cholesterol levels and overwhelming preponderance of the large HDL subfractions (32).

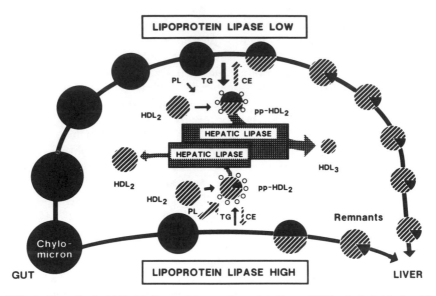

FIG. 1. The effect of TG-rich lipoproteins on the catabolism of HDL$_2$. In individuals with high lipoprotein lipase activity, postprandial TG-rich lipoproteins do not accumulate in the blood. Surface components, predominantly phospholipids (open circles), are rapidly liberated from TG-rich lipoproteins and assimilated by HDL$_2$. Hepatic lipase hydrolyzes phospholipids from these pp HDL$_2$ and thus restores the phospholipid acceptor function of HDL$_2$ for renewed postprandial lipemia. In this situation, HDL$_2$ levels are not reduced in the steady state. By contrast, when lipoprotein lipase activity is low or partially saturated by lipoproteins carrying endogenous triglycerides, increased amounts of postprandial TG-rich lipoproteins accumulate and circulate for a prolonged time. This allows for an extensive exchange of chylomicron–TG (black areas) and HDL$_2$–cholesteryl esters (shaded areas) mediated by LTP-I. Hepatic lipase now removes not only phospholipids from the surface of pp HDL$_2$, but also triglycerides from their core. HDL$_2$ are converted to smaller HDL$_3$, and the steady-state levels of HDL$_2$ decrease. From ref. 15.

When LTP-I is present in the blood, the amount of triglyceride transferred to HDL depends on the rate of the LTP-I reaction. The rate is a function of the concentration of TG-rich donor lipoproteins (6), and the overall reaction also depends on the time available for exchange. Clearly, postprandial lipemia—which shows great variations even in normolipidemic individuals (15,20,29)—can both allow and restrict the operation of these variables (Fig. 1).

Triglycerides and the Formation of HDL$_2$

Unlike chylomicrons or very low-density lipoproteins (VLDL), HDL are not released into the circulation as mature spherical lipoproteins. The secretory precursors of HDL are discoidal micellar complexes of apolipoproteins, phospholipids, and unesterified cholesterol. They are synthesized by liver (33) and intestine (34) and mature in the vascular compartment, where LCAT generates hydrophobic cholesteryl esters to form a spherical HDL core (35,36).

The biosynthetic rate of apoA-I, the major protein component of HDL, is one determinant of HDL plasma levels: (i) HDL concentrations are extremely low in the blood of patients homozygous for familial apoA-I/apoC-III deficiency and one-half of normal in obligate heterozygotes (37). The deficiency is caused by a DNA inversion that results in a reciprocal fusion of the apoA-I and apoC-III gene transcriptional units (38). (ii) Overexpression of human apoA-I in transgenic mice correlates with an increase in HDL–cholesterol. However, the elevation is confined to small, dense particles such as human HDL_3 (39). These results clearly indicate that, while apoA-I is necessary for HDL particles to exist, at least one additional factor must be critical for the formation of HDL_2.

We suggest that this factor is the catabolic rate of TG-rich lipoproteins. Hydrolysis of the triglyceride moiety of these particles by lipoprotein lipase liberates an excess of surface components, particularly phospholipids that are transferred to the HDL fraction, within which they promote the formation of larger, more lipid-rich, less dense particles. This was unambiguously demonstrated in an *in vitro* lipolysis system containing human TG-rich lipoproteins, HDL_3, and purified bovine milk lipoprotein lipase: As lipolysis took place, HDL_3 assimilated surface components of the lipolyzed TG-rich lipoproteins and assumed density and flotation characteristics of HDL_2 (40).

Conditions, however, might be different *in vivo:* First, the gradients directing the flux of phospholipids from TG-rich lipoproteins under lipolysis to HDL are probably smaller than those generated *in vitro*. Second, other lipoproteins and membranes will compete with preexisting HDL_3 for incorporating the surface components. Finally, the capacity of HDL to accept phospholipids is limited by the compressibility of the particles' surface monolayer (41,42). Considering the intravascular half-life of chylomicron triglycerides to be on the order of 5 min (43,44), phospholipids derived from these lipoproteins will surge quickly in the postprandial state and will have to be assimilated before a significant enlargement of the core of a spherical HDL_3 by the action of LCAT can occur. These factors seem to work together to keep the phospholipid enrichment of pp HDL_3 (45) far below the requirements for a direct conversion of HDL_3 to HDL_2.

We therefore investigated *in vitro* whether an additional structure would be necessary to temporarily accommodate TG-rich lipoprotein-derived phospholipids for the eventual anabolic formation of HDL_2 from smaller precursors. This was indeed the case: Only when discoidal HDL in addition to spherical HDL_3 were exposed to TG-rich lipoproteins undergoing lipolysis, an HDL subfraction was formed that displayed density, size, and composition of native HDL_2. Like native HDL_2, these product particles were stable in the presence of HDL_3 and cell membranes. By contrast, when no lipolysis took place in this system, a simple adduct of spherical HDL_3 and discoidal HDL was formed which was distinctly different from native HDL_2 and HDL_3 (G. Miesenböck and J. R. Patsch, manuscript in preparation). Hence, whether an HDL precur-

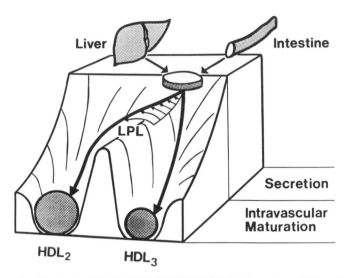

FIG. 2. The role of lipolysis of TG-RICH LIPOPROTEINS in the formation of HDL_2. Mature spherical HDL are present in the blood as two thermodynamically stable forms, i.e., HDL_2 and HDL_3. They are, however, not secreted as such: Liver and intestine synthesize discoidal precursors consisting of surface lipids, but devoid of core lipids. Apolipoproteins are located at the perimeter of these discs. Within the vascular compartment, the discoidal precursors are transformed into spherical HDL by the action of LCAT, providing the core lipids (illustrated as the path leading from the disc to HDL_3). Transformation of the discoidal precursor into HDL_2 is also possible. This requires the simultaneous action of lipoprotein lipase (LPL) on TG-rich lipoproteins, supplying additional surface components.

sor enters the HDL_2 pool or the HDL_3 pool is not decided for a particle once it has attained the mature spherical structure but earlier, during the process of maturation from the discoidal to the spherical shape. Again, the driving force that directs a maturing discoidal HDL into the HDL_2 pool is lipolysis of TG-rich lipoproteins (Fig. 2).

CONCLUSION

In the present article, we have delineated that the tight inverse relationship between triglycerides and HDL–cholesterol is caused by the influence that the metabolism of TG-rich lipoproteins exerts on HDL. This opens the possibility that the very powerful negative association of HDL–cholesterol and CAD is in reality a positive relationship between CAD and TG-rich lipoproteins or some of their subfractions. In the Helsinki Heart Study, cardiac end points were reduced to a considerably larger extent than was expected from the lowering of LDL–cholesterol by administration of gemfibrozil (4). This additional reduction has been ascribed to the simultaneous rise of HDL–cholesterol. However, it may be of significance that those individuals benefited most from the intervention who experienced the most pronounced reduction in triglycerides (46).

From the evidence we have provided in our discussion, the HDL–cholesterol level obtained in a given subject at a given time point represents an integral for triglyceride transport extending back about 1 week (see Fig. 3 in ref. 20). Thus, it is not surprising that such an integrative parameter eliminates triglycerides as a risk factor for CAD in epidemiologic studies employing multivariate analysis (19,47). In this context, glycosylated hemoglobin (HbA_{1c}) comes to mind, which has generally been accepted as an extremely valuable integrative clinical parameter to estimate glycemic control for the preceding 6-week period (48). Although epidemiologic evidence is not available at this time, one can reasonably anticipate the correlation of HbA_{1c} to late diabetic complications to be superior to that of single blood glucose measurements. This superiority of HbA_{1c} as a correlate to late complications would by no means qualify it as a more likely causative agent than elevated glucose levels. It is quite possible that HDL–cholesterol is for triglycerides what HbA_{1c} is for glucose. If this is true, then deranged triglyceride transport is the cause for CAD, and HDL is the indicator.

ACKNOWLEDGMENT

The work of the authors discussed in this article was supported by grant HL-27341 from the National Institutes of Health and by grant S-46/06 from the Austrian "Fonds zur Förderung der wissenschaftlichen Forschung."

REFERENCES

1. Rhoads GG, Gulbrandsen GL, Kagan A. Serum lipoproteins and coronary heart disease in a population study of Hawaii Japanese men. *N Engl J Med* 1976;294:293–298.
2. Gordon T, Castelli WP, Hjortland MC, Kannel WB, Dawber TR. High density lipoprotein as a protective factor against coronary heart disease. *Am J Med* 1977;62:707–714.
3. Tyroler HA. Epidemiology of plasma high-density lipoprotein cholesterol levels. *Circulation* 1980;62(Suppl IV):IV-1–IV-3.
4. Frick MH, Elo O, Haapa K, et al. Helsinki Heart Study: primary-prevention trial with gemfibrozil in middle-aged men with dyslipidemia. *N Engl J Med* 1987;317:1237–1245.
5. Glomset JA. The plasma lecithin:cholesterol acyltransferase reaction. *J Lipid Res* 1968;9:155–167.
6. Morton RE, Zilversmit DB. Inter-relationship of lipids transferred by the lipid-transfer protein isolated from human lipoprotein-deficient plasma. *J Biol Chem* 1983;258:11751–11757.
7. Albers JJ, Tollefson JH, Chen C-H, Steinmetz A. Isolation and characterization of human plasma lipid transfer proteins. *Arteriosclerosis* 1984;4:49–58.
8. Brown MS, Goldstein JL. A receptor-mediated pathway for cholesterol homeostasis. *Science* 1986;232:34–47.
9. Havel RJ. Functional activities of hepatic lipoprotein receptors. *Annu Rev Physiol* 1986;48:119–134.
10. Koo C, Innerarity TL, Mahley RW. Obligatory role of cholesterol and apolipoprotein E in the formation of large cholesterol-enriched and receptor-active high density lipoproteins. *J Biol Chem* 1985;260:11934–11943.
11. DeLalla OF, Gofman JW. Ultracentrifugal analysis of serum lipoproteins. *Methods Biochem Anal* 1954;1:459–478.

12. Patsch JR, Sailer S, Kostner G, Sandhofer F, Holasek A, Braunsteiner H. Separation of the main lipoprotein density classes from human plasma by rate-zonal ultracentrifugation. *J Lipid Res* 1974;15:356–366.
13. Patsch W, Schonfeld G, Gotto AM Jr, Patsch JR. Characterization of human high density lipoproteins by zonal ultracentrifugation. *J Biol Chem* 1980;255:3178–3185.
14. Anderson DA, Nichols AV, Pan SS, Lindgren FT. High density lipoprotein distribution. Resolution and determination of three major components in a normal population sample. *Atherosclerosis* 1978;29:161–179.
15. Patsch JR, Prasad S, Gotto AM Jr, Patsch W. High density lipoprotein$_2$. Relationship of the plasma levels of this lipoprotein species to its composition, to the magnitude of postprandial lipemia, and to the activities of lipoprotein lipase and hepatic lipase. *J Clin Invest* 1987;80:341–347.
16. Miller NE, Hammett F, Saltissi S, van Zeller H, Coltart J, Lewis B. Relation of angiographically defined coronary artery disease to plasma lipoprotein subfractions and apolipoproteins. *Br Med J* 1981;282:1741–1744.
17. Ballantyne FC, Clark RS, Simpson HS, Ballantyne D. High density and low density lipoprotein subfractions in survivors of myocardial infarction and in control subjects. *Metabolism* 1982;31:433–437.
18. Gofman JW, DeLalla O, Glazier F, et al. Serum lipoprotein transport system in health, metabolic disorders, atherosclerosis, and coronary heart disease. *Plasma* 1954;2:413–484.
19. Castelli WP, Doyle JT, Gordon T, et al. HDL cholesterol and other lipids in coronary heart disease. The cooperative lipoprotein phenotyping study. *Circulation* 1977;55:767–772.
20. Patsch JR, Karlin JB, Scott LW, Smith LC, Gotto AM Jr. Inverse relationship between blood levels of high density lipoprotein subfraction 2 and magnitude of postprandial lipemia. *Proc Natl Acad Sci USA* 1983;80:1449–1453.
21. Nilsson-Ehle P, Garfinkel AS, Schotz MC. Lipolytic enzymes and plasma lipoprotein metabolism. *Annu Rev Biochem* 1980;49:667–693.
22. Jackson RL. Lipoprotein lipase and hepatic lipase. In: Boyer PD, ed. *The enzymes,* Vol. XVI. New York: Academic Press, 1983:141–181.
23. Olivecrona T, Bengtsson-Olivecrona G. Heparin and lipases. In: Lane DA, Lindahl U, eds. *Heparin.* London: Edward Arnold, 1989:335–361.
24. Kuusi T, Saarinen P, Nikkilä EA. Evidence for the role of hepatic endothelial lipase in the metabolism of plasma high density lipoprotein$_2$ in man. *Atherosclerosis* 1980;36:589–593.
25. Nikkilä EA, Taskinen M-R, Kekki M. Relation of plasma high-density lipoprotein cholesterol to lipoprotein-lipase activity in adipose tissue and skeletal muscle of man. *Atherosclerosis* 1978;29:497–501.
26. Brown MS, Goldstein JL. Drugs used in the treatment of hyperlipoproteinemias. In: Gilman AG, Goodman LS, Rall TW, Murad F, eds. *The pharmacological basis of therapeutics,* 7th edition. New York: Macmillan, 1985:827–845.
27. Breckenridge WC, Little JA, Alaupovic P, et al. Lipoprotein abnormalities associated with a familial deficiency of hepatic lipase. *Atherosclerosis* 1982;45:161–179.
28. Demant T, Carlson LA, Holmquist L, et al. Lipoprotein metabolism in hepatic lipase deficiency: studies on the turnover of apolipoprotein B and on the effect of hepatic lipase on high density lipoprotein. *J Lipid Res* 1988;29:1603–1611.
29. Patsch JR, Prasad S, Gotto AM Jr, Bengtsson-Olivecrona G. Postprandial lipemia: a key for the conversion of high density lipoprotein$_2$ into high density lipoprotein$_3$ by hepatic lipase. *J Clin Invest* 1984;74:2017–2023.
30. Kuusi T, Kinnunen PKJ, Nikkilä EA. Hepatic endothelial lipase antiserum influences rat plasma low and high density lipoproteins in vivo. *FEBS Lett* 1979;104:384–388.
31. Grosser J, Schrecker O, Greten H. Function of hepatic triglyceride lipase in lipoprotein metabolism. *J Lipid Res* 1981;22:437–442.
32. Brown ML, Inazu A, Hesler CB, et al. Molecular basis of lipid transfer protein deficiency in a family with increased high-density lipoproteins. *Nature (Lond)* 1989;342:448–451.
33. Hamilton RL, Williams MC, Fielding CJ, Havel RJ. Discoidal bilayer structure of nascent high density lipoproteins from perfused rat liver. *J Clin Invest* 1976;58:667–680.
34. Green PHR, Tall AR, Glickman RM. Rat intestine secretes discoid high density lipoprotein. *J Clin Invest* 1978;61:528–534.

35. Glomset JA, Norum KR. The metabolic role of lecithin:cholesterol acyltransferase: perspectives from pathology. *Adv Lipid Res* 1973;11:1–65.
36. Matz CE, Jonas A. Reaction of human lecithin cholesterol acyltransferase with synthetic micellar complexes of apolipoprotein A-I, phosphatidylcholine, and cholesterol. *J Biol Chem* 1982;257:4541–4546.
37. Norum RA, Lakier JB, Goldstein S, et al. Familial deficiency of apolipoproteins A-I and C-III and precocious coronary-artery disease. *N Engl J Med* 1982;306:1513–1519.
38. Karathanasis SK, Ferris E, Haddad IA. DNA inversion within the apolipoproteins AI/CIII/AIV-encoding gene cluster of certain patients with premature atherosclerosis. *Proc Natl Acad Sci USA* 1987;84:7198–7202.
39. Walsh A, Ito Y, Breslow JL. High levels of human apolipoprotein A-I in transgenic mice result in increased plasma levels of small high density lipoprotein (HDL) particles comparable to human HDL_3. *J Biol Chem* 1989;264:6488–6494.
40. Patsch JR, Gotto AM Jr, Olivecrona T, Eisenberg S. Formation of high density lipoprotein$_2$-like particles during lipolysis of very low density lipoproteins in vitro. *Proc Natl Acad Sci USA* 1978;75:4519–4523.
41. Shen BW, Scanu AM, Kezdy FJ. Structure of human serum lipoproteins inferred from compositional analysis. *Proc Natl Acad Sci USA* 1977;74:837–841.
42. Ibdah JA, Lund-Katz S, Phillips MC. Molecular packing of high-density and low-density lipoprotein surface lipids and apolipoprotein A-I binding. *Biochemistry* 1989;28:1126–1133.
43. Nestel PJ. Relationship between plasma triglycerides and removal of chylomicrons. *J Clin Invest* 1964;43:943–949.
44. Grundy SM, Mok HYI. Chylomicron clearance in normal and hyperlipidemic man. *Metabolism* 1976;25:1225–1239.
45. Tall AR, Blum CB, Forester GP, Nelson CA. Changes in the distribution and composition of plasma high density lipoproteins after ingestion of fat. *J Biol Chem* 1982;257:198–207.
46. Manninen V, Elo MO, Frick MH, et al. Lipid alterations and decline in the incidence of coronary heart disease in the Helsinki Heart Study. *JAMA* 1988;260:641–651.
47. Hulley SB, Rosenman RH, Bawol RD, Brand RJ, Epidemiology as a guide to clinical decisions: the association between triglyceride and coronary heart disease. *N Engl J Med* 1980;302:1383–1389.
48. Unger RH, Foster DW. Diabetes mellitus. In: Wilson JD, Foster DW, eds. *Williams' textbook of endocrinology,* 7th edition. Philadelphia: Saunders, 1985:1018–1080.

Atherosclerosis Reviews, Volume 21,
edited by A. Leaf and P. C. Weber.
Raven Press, Ltd., New York © 1990.

Lipid-Lowering Drugs and Atherosclerosis

Josef R. Patsch

*Division of Clinical Atherosclerosis Research, Department of Medicine,
University of Innsbruck, A-6020 Innsbruck, Austria*

A number of clinical trials completed in recent years provide evidence that a modification of blood lipids toward normal will reduce the risk of atherosclerosis. The National Institutes of Health (NIH) Consensus Development Conference on Lowering Blood Cholesterol to Prevent Heart Disease (1) recommended that Americans at risk of coronary artery disease (CAD) be treated aggressively with diet and, when necessary, with drugs. The National Cholesterol Education Program (NCEP) (2) and the European Atherosclerosis Society (3) have provided guidelines for the evaluation of adults and for the institution of therapies with either diet alone or diet and drugs (Table 1).

Treatment always has to begin with diet. If the patient is overweight, caloric restriction is necessary. To lower elevated cholesterol levels, a stepwise approach, as recommended by the American Heart Association (4), should be adopted. If diet does not accomplish the desired reduction of plasma cholesterol, drug therapy should be considered. The drugs used to lower blood lipids, their clinical use, their dosage, and adverse effects are shown in Table 2.

Selection of a lipid-lowering drug is based on lipoprotein analysis from plasma. Different groups of lipid-lowering drugs have different effects on very-low-density lipoprotein (VLDL), remnants, low-density lipoprotein (LDL), and high-density lipoprotein (HDL). Because of the often necessary long-term use of lipid-lowering drugs, patients must be monitored at regular intervals not only for blood lipids but also for side effects.

The bile acid sequestrants cholestyramine and colestipol are not absorbed, but bind bile acids in the intestine interrupting their enterohepatic circulation. As a result, bile acids are excreted, cholesterol absorption decreases slightly, hepatic bile acid synthesis from cholesterol increases, and hepatocellular cholesterol levels decrease. This leads to an enhanced expression of LDL receptors on the surface of hepatocytes and increases the removal of LDL by the liver. Because of the effects on cellular cholesterol synthesis, bile acid sequestrants tend to increase hepatic VLDL production with a possible rise in plasma triglycerides.

Nicotinic acid effectively lowers VLDL, intermediate-density lipoprotein (IDL), and LDL via reduced VLDL production, which is associated with in-

TABLE 1. *National cholesterol education program guidelines*

Serum cholesterol level	Degree of risk	Recommendation
<200 mg/dl	Low	Recheck cholesterol every 5 years
200–239 mg/dl without CAD or other risk factors[a]	Borderline high	Restrict dietary saturated fat, cholesterol, and calories, if overweight Recheck cholesterol annually Lipoprotein profile[b] with CAD or at least two other risk factors
200–230 mg/dl with CAD or at least two other risk factors[a]	High	Obtain lipoprotein profile[b] Begin with diet and make maximal efforts to reach desirable LDL cholesterol by nonpharmacological means If LDL cholesterol remains >190 mg/dl after diet, definitely prescribe drugs
≥240 mg/dl	High	Same as above

Adapted from ref. 2.

[a] Risk factors include HDL cholesterol < 35 mg/dl, male sex, family history of early CAD, cigarette smoking, hypertension, diabetes mellitus, and >30% overweight.

[b] Once lipoprotein profile is required, decision-making should shift from total serum cholesterol to LDL cholesterol. Treatment is based on the concentration of serum LDL cholesterol: <130 mg/dl, desirable range; 130 to 159 mg/dl, borderline high risk; >160 mg/dl, high risk.

creases in HDL, particularly in HDL_2. The drug inhibits the mobilization of free fatty acids from adipose tissue and decreases esterification of fatty acids in the liver which both contribute to reduced VLDL production. The lipid-lowering action is not related to its role as coenzyme. Nicotinic acid has been demonstrated to reduce the mortality from CAD (5). Side effects are cutaneous flushing, dry skin, nausea, vomiting, diarrhea, increases in uric acid and blood sugar levels, and liver function abnormalities. In the coronary drug project, the drug was associated with an increased prevalence of atrial fibrillation. Because of its side effects, nicotinic acid should be used only in high-risk hyperlipoproteinemic patients in whom other drug regimens are insufficient or their use is not possible.

Clofibrate lowers triglycerides and cholesterol by accelerating the intravascular catabolism of VLDL and increasing cholesterol excretion into the bile. The World Health Organization (WHO) Primary Prevention Trial (6) demonstrated that treatment of hypercholesterolemic patients with clofibrate was associated with a higher noncardiac mortality, which was mainly due to an increased incidence of malignant neoplasms and complications of cholecystectomy. Clofibrate has been associated with cardiac arrhythmias, cardiomegaly, angina, claudication, acute myositis, and thromboembolic phenomena. Milder side effects include gastrointestinal disturbances, weight gain, drowsiness, weakness, skin rash, and alopecia. Clofibrate enhances also the effects of phenytoin and tolbutamide. Because of its serious side effects, use of clofibrate should be reserved only for certain patients with type III hyperlipoproteinemia.

TABLE 2. *Summary of lipid-lowering drugs*

Agents	Clinical use (elevation of lipoprotein)	Side effects	Daily dosage (range)
Cholestyramine Colestipol	LDL	Constipation, bloating Can alter absorption of other drugs Can increase triglyceride levels Hyperchloremic acidosis (rare) Hypoprothrombinemia	12–24 g 15–30 g
Nicotinic acid	VLDL, remnants, LDL	Altered liver function, increased uric acid, hyperglycemia, cutaneous flushing, gastrointestinal upset, hyperpigmentation	3–6 g
Clofibrate	VLDL, remnants, LDL	Altered liver function, myositis, increased incidence of cholelithiasis and perhaps gastrointestinal malignancies, potentiation of warfarin, impotence, skin rash, cardiac arrhythmias, thrombembolic phenomena	1–2 g
Gemfibrozil	VLDL, remnants, LDL	Nausea, diarrhea, myositis, skin rash, eosinophilia, potentiation of anticoagulants, mild hyperglycemic effect	1,200 mg
Probucol	LDL	Gastrointestinal upset, prolongs QT interval, may increase ventricular irritability, lowers HDL cholesterol (significance of this is unknown)	1 g
Lovastatin	LDL	Altered liver functions at 3 to 10 months, myolysis	20–80 mg

Gemfibrozil lowers VLDL mainly by an inhibition of VLDL production and by enhanced catabolism of VLDL. Reductions of LDL are moderate, but HDL often increase. In the Helsinki Heart Study (HHS), gemfibrozil reduced plasma triglycerides by 35%, decreased LDL cholesterol by about 8% and increased HDL cholesterol by 9% (7). When compared with the placebo group, the incidence of CAD was reduced by 34%. When compared with the results from the Lipid Research Clinics Primary Prevention Trial (LRC-CPPT) (8), percentage lowering of cholesterol in the Helsinki Heart Study was two times more effective in the prevention of definite cardiac end points. This difference has been attributed to a distinct effect of gemfibrozil on HDL cholesterol and plasma triglycerides. Unlike its congener clofibrate in the WHO study, gemfibrozil did not increase the noncardiac mortality due to cancer in the HHS.

Other fibric acid derivatives not available in the U.S. are fenofibrate and bezafibrate, which are used widely in Europe and elsewhere. At their recommended doses of 300 mg and 600 mg/day they appear to have effects on blood lipids comparable to that of gemfibrozil. With respect to their side-effect profile, they may be distinguished with less gastrointestinal upset but with more skin rash.

Probucol is moderately effective in lowering LDL cholesterol and also reduces HDL cholesterol (9). Studies in the WHHL rabbit suggest that probucol may reduce the rate of lesion formation independent of its effect on plasma cholesterol. A lipophilic antioxidant, the drug inhibits oxidation of LDL *in vitro* and may enhance removal of LDL by sites other than the LDL receptor. Only 2% to 10% of the very lipid-soluble drug is absorbed and the drug tends to accumulate in adipose tissue, where it can be found months after discontinuance. Because of this and because the safety of probucol has not been established in children or in pregnant women, it has been recommended that women discontinue probucol and use birth control measures for at least 6 months before attempting to become pregnant.

Lovastatin is the first approved drug of a group of agents that competitively inhibit 3 hydroxy-3-methylglutaryl coenzyme A (HMG-CoA) reductase (10). The primary effect of the drug is to inhibit endogenous cholesterol synthesis and to reduce cellular cholesterol. Consequently, expression of LDL receptors is increased. To be effective, HMG-CoA-reductase inhibitors require at least one normal LDL receptor allele, whose transcriptional activity can be enhanced by a depletion of cellular cholesterol. Rhabdomyolysis is a potentially serious side effect in patients receiving cyclosporin after organ transplants. Other HMG-CoA-reductase inhibitors not currently available in the U.S. include pravastatin and simvastatin.

D-Thyroxine reduces plasma cholesterol by enhancing LDL removal via up-regulated LDL-receptor activity. In the coronary drug project (5), D-thyroxine was withdrawn from the study because of increased coronary and other cardiovascular mortality, as well as nonfatal myocardial infarctions. Therefore, the usefulness of the drug is extremely limited, particularly in patients with CAD.

Additional drugs used occasionally to lower plasma lipids include neomycin and sitosterol. However, these two agents are not approved by the Food and Drug Administration for reducing plasma cholesterol, triglycerides, or lipoproteins.

Combination Drug Therapy

Two major advantages of combining two hypolipidemic drugs with different mechanisms of action are that (a) they can be more effective than single hypolipidemic agents and (b) they can have fewer side effects because two drugs are used at doses much lower than the maximum dose of each drug where respective side effects are more likely to occur. Most effective combination therapies include usually a bile acid sequestrant. For instance, low doses of cholestyramine (4 to 8 g/day) combined with low doses of either nicotinic acid (1.5 g/day) or HMG-CoA-reductase inhibitor (Lovastatin 20 mg/day) can be both well tolerated and very effective in reducing LDL and raising HDL cholesterol levels. However, other combination therapies appear to have an unfavorable side-effect profile;

combinations of HMG-CoA-reductase inhibitors with either nicotinic acid or gemfibrozil have been associated with rhabdomyolysis.

In summary, there exists clear evidence provided by large clinical trials (7,8) that in individuals with elevated blood lipids the use of lipid-lowering drugs will reduce the risk of atherosclerosis. With this evidence and clear guidelines for patient evaluation and therapy (2,3), appropriate diet and judicious use of lipid-lowering drugs should help to widely combat atherosclerosis in patients with elevated blood lipids. Also, from the very active ongoing research into the pathophysiology of lipid transport one can expect development of additional effective and safe lipid-lowering agents.

REFERENCES

1. Consensus Conference. Lowering blood cholesterol to prevent heart disease. *JAMA* 1985;253: 2080–2086.
2. The Expert Panel. Report of the national cholesterol education program. Expert panel on detection, evaluation, and treatment of high blood cholesterol in adults. *Arch Intern Med* 1988;148: 36–69.
3. Study Group, European Atherosclerosis Society. The recognition and management of hyperlipidemia in adults. A policy statement of the European Atherosclerosis Society. *Eur Heart J* 1988;9:571–600.
4. AHA Special Report. Recommendations for treatment of hyperlipidemia in adults. A joint statement of the nutrition committee and the council on atherosclerosis. *Circulation* 1984;69: 1065A–1090A.
5. Canner PL, Berge KG, Wenger NK, et al. Fifteen year mortality in coronary drug project patients: long-term benefits with niacin. *J Am Coll Cardiol* 1986;8:1245–1255.
6. Committee of Principal Investigators. WHO cooperative trial on primary prevention of ischemic heart disease using clofibrate to lower serum cholesterol: mortality follow-up. *Lancet* 1980;2:379–385.
7. Frick MH, Elo O, Haapa K, et al. Helsinki Heart Study: primary prevention trial with gemfibrozil in middle-aged men with dyslipidemia. *N Engl J Med* 1987;317:1237–1245.
8. Lipid Research Clinics Program. The lipid research clinics coronary primary prevention trial. I. Reduction in incidence of coronary heart disease. *JAMA* 1984;251:351–364.
9. Illingworth DR. Lipid-lowering drugs. An overview of indications and optimum therapeutic use. *Drugs* 1987;33:259–279.
10. Alberts AW, Chen J, Kuron G, et al. Mevinolin, a highly potent competitive inhibitor of HMG-CoA reductase and cholesterol lowering agent. *Proc Natl Acad Sci USA* 1980;77:3957–3961.

Atherosclerosis Reviews, Volume 21,
edited by A. Leaf and P. C. Weber.
Raven Press, Ltd., New York © 1990.

The Effects on Coronary Artery Disease of Treatment for Mild Hypertension

W. E. Miall

Sidegarth, Staveley, Kendal, Cumbria LA8 9NN, England

The recently completed trials of drug treatment for mild hypertension showed important benefits for stroke but no overall benefit for coronary artery disease (CAD). In addition, the blood pressures of those receiving active treatment were controlled at lower levels, and this reduced the progression from mild to severe hypertension and postponed the onset of the vascular complications of the severe disease.

Epidemiological studies have shown the relationship between stroke and hypertension to be closer than that between CAD and hypertension. Control of blood pressure would be expected to have a more direct and immediate effect on Charcot–Bouchard aneurysms than it would on the intimal plaques and thromboses in the larger vessels. For purely pathological reasons, we might expect control of hypertension to result in a greater reduction in stroke than in CAD, but several other explanations for the difference between the stroke and coronary results have been suggested.

Even the larger trials were too small to detect what would be a major public health benefit—i.e., a 10% to 15% reduction in hypertension-related events. MacMahon et al. (1) calculate that even after pooling all the major trials, the sample size would be insufficient for detecting such a modest albeit potentially important reduction in CAD events. Perhaps the trials were too short in duration—their average length was 5.6 years. Many factors influence the incidence of CAD, and the control for 5 or 6 years of just one of them, hypertension, may have been insufficient to modify significantly a chronic disease that may have been developing for most of a lifetime.

Thiazide diuretics formed the basis of treatment in all the trials. The metabolic changes associated with the use of thiazides may have counteracted what benefit would have been expected from the blood pressure reduction. Such biochemical changes involve the shifting of the distributions of serum electrolytes (including potassium and magnesium, which may have influenced the frequency of cardiac arrhythmias and sudden deaths) and of serum uric acid, serum lipids, and blood glucose in directions that favor the development of CAD.

Further trials will be needed to assess the value of newer antihypertensive drugs; calcium antagonists and converting enzyme inhibitors, for example, have not yet been subjected to the rigorous testing applied to thiazide diuretics and β-blocking agents. The use of placebo treatment may be considered unjustifiable in future trials that attempt to measure the effects on such hard end points as deaths, strokes, and myocardial infarctions. If new trials are designed to measure minor differences between the protection conferred by a new drug over that conferred by its predecessor, either very large numbers of participants or less stringent end-point criteria will be required. In addition, any such trials will need to compare the benefits of new drugs with those of thiazides and β-blockers. New trials would provide opportunities to answer some of the still outstanding questions raised by the previous studies.

This paper draws attention to some of these questions, illustrating largely from the Medical Research Council's treatment trial for mild hypertension, which was the only study designed to be able to compare thiazide treatment with β-blocker treatment, and to compare each with a placebo-treated control group (2–4).

TABLE 1. *The larger randomized treatment trials for hypertension*

Trial	No. of subjects	Age (yr)	DBP(V) range	Sex	Active drugs	Control group
VA[a]	380	Mean 52	90–114	M	Hydrochlorothiazide reserpine, hydrallazine	Placebo
USPHS	389	21–55	90–114	M, F	Chlorothiazide	Placebo
Oslo	785	40–49	<110, DBP $\geq$95 or SBP $\geq$150	M	Hydrochlorothiazide	No treatment
ANBPS	3,427	30–69	95–109	M, F	Chlorothiazide	Placebo
MRC	17,354	35–64	90–109	M, F	Bendrofluazide or propranolol	Placebo
HDFP[b]	7,825	30–69	90–104	M, F	Chlorothalidone, hydrochlorothiazide, reserpine methyl-dopa	Referred care
MRFIT	8,012	35–57	90–114	M	Chlorothalidone, hydrochlorothiazide	Usual care
IPPPSH	6,357	40–64	100–125	M, F	Oxyprenolol	Placebo or non-β-blocker therapy
HAPPHY	6,569	40–64	100–130	M	Bendrofluazide or hydrochlorothiazide	Atenolol or metoprolol

Note: DBP = diastolic blood pressure; VA = Veterans Administration; USPHS = U.S. Public Health Service; SBP = systolic blood pressure. See text for further abbreviations.
[a] Part 2.
[b] Stratum 1.

CAD MORBIDITY AND MORTALITY IN THE TRIALS

Five major placebo- (or no-treatment) controlled trials for mild hypertension were carried out (Table 1). Each trial included predominantly middle-aged adults with diastolic Korotkoff phase V pressures confirmed in the 90 to 109 mm Hg range. [Details of their designs are described elsewhere (2,5–8).] Two nonplacebo-controlled trials, the U.S. Hypertension Detection and Follow-up Program (HDFP) (9) and the Multiple Risk Factor Intervention Trial (MRFIT) (10), compared a stepped-care form of treatment with referral back to a usual source of care. Neither of these is comparable with the studies in which control subjects were untreated; they were designed to answer quite different questions, but much of the data they produced is highly relevant to any discussion of the effects of antihypertensive treatment on CAD end points. Two studies, the Heart Attack Primary Prevention in Hypertension trial (HAPPHY) (11) and the International Prospective Primary Prevention Study in Hypertension (IPP-PSH) (12), compared therapy with different classes of drugs but without an untreated control group; neither was restricted to mild hypertension. The trial conducted by the European Working Party for Hypertension in the Elderly (EWPHE) (13) recruited patients over the age of 60 years, some of whom had severe disease; it is not included in this review.

None of the five trials with untreated controls showed any overall effect on coronary end points (Table 2). In the Veterans Administration trial and Australian National Blood Pressure Study (ANBPS) fatal myocardial infarction (MI) was less frequent in treated than it was in control subjects but was balanced by higher numbers of nonfatal events among treated than it was among control

TABLE 2. *The effects of treatment of mild hypertension on CAD events in various trials*

Trial	Sudden deaths or fatal MI		Nonfatal CAD events		Total	
	Treated	Controls	Treated	Controls	Treated	Controls
Placebo-controlled trials						
Veterans Administration[a]	4	8	7	5	11	13
USPHS	1	1	7	6	8	7
Oslo	6	2	8	8	14	10
ANBPS	5	11	28	22	33	33
MRC	106	97	116	137	222	234
Total	122	119	166	178	288	297
Nonplacebo-controlled trials						
HDFP[b]	30	56				
MRFIT[c]	80	79				
Total	110	135				

Note: Abbreviations as in Table 1.
[a] Part 2.
[b] Stratum 1.
[c] Hypertensives.

TABLE 3. *All coronary events and rates/1,000 person-years of observation, according to age, sex, and randomized treatment regimens*

| Sex | Age | Treated | | | | | | Controls | |
| | | Bendrofluazide | | Propranolol | | Active drugs[b] | | Placebo | |
		N	Rate	N	Rate	N	Rate	N	Rate
Male	35–44	11	4.4	10	3.9	21	4.2	17	3.3
	45–54	33	6.9	39	8.0	72	7.5	83	8.7
	55–64	55	14.9	36	9.6	91	12.2	100	13.4
	Total[a]	99	9.0	85	7.6	184	8.3	200	9.0
Female	35–44	1	0.6	1	0.6	2	0.6	1	0.3
	45–54	7	1.7	5	1.2	12	1.4	9	1.1
	55–64	12	2.6	12	2.6	24	2.6	24	2.6
	Total[a]	20	1.9	18	1.7	38	1.8	34	1.7
Both	Total[a]	119	5.6	103	4.8	222	5.2	234	5.4

From ref. 4.
[a] Age-adjusted rates.
[b] Those randomized to either bendrofluazide or propranolol.

subjects. The Oslo trial and the Medical Research Council (MRC) trial showed nonsignificant excesses of fatal events in treated subjects. Overall, there were 288 CAD events in the treated groups and 297 among controls.

In Stratum 1 of HDFP (with diastolic pressures of 90–104 mm Hg) there was an impressive 46% reduction in fatal MI (ICD 410) in the more actively treated stepped-care group. The meaning of this finding, which conflicts with the results in all other studies, is not clear. For other ischemic heart disease deaths (ICD 411–413) in the HDFP the trend was reversed, resulting in an overall 19% reduction in fatal CAD in the stepped-care group. The HDFP was designed to provide comparable mortality data for stepped-care and referred-care groups, but it was recognized that morbidity comparisons would be open to various forms of bias. In the hypertensive section of the MRFIT, fatal MI occurred with equal frequency in the special-care and usual-care groups.

In the MRC trial, the influence of the trial drugs, bendrofluazide and propranolol, on fatal and nonfatal coronary events, on sudden deaths, and on the ECG changes of MI were examined. When compared with untreated controls, the two active drug groups often showed opposing trends, with the β-blocker tending to show benefit and the thiazide tending to show an adverse effect. For fatal CAD events, the β-blocker showed a 5% reduction and the thiazide showed a nonsignificant 22% excess. For all fatal and nonfatal CAD events, the results in the two drug groups did not differ significantly, nor did those between each drug group and the placebo group (Table 3).

The MRC trial had been monitored by sequential analysis from its outset (4). The sequential plot showing the accumulation of CAD events among all treated and all control subjects (Fig. 1) never approached the 5% or 1% boundaries corresponding to significant differences between the two groups. The plot for

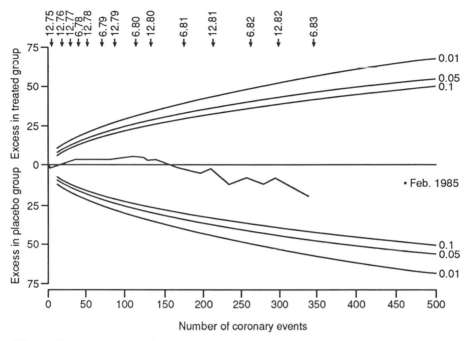

FIG. 1. MRC treatment trial for mild hypertension. Sequential chart for coronary events (both sexes); treated vs. control subjects. From ref. 4.

events among men receiving the two active drugs (Fig. 2) had twice reached the 5% significance boundary, suggesting less protection by bendrofluazide (which was given in a dose of 5 mg b.i.d.) than by propranolol (given in a dose of up to 160 mg b.i.d.). This observation was made at a time when the incidence of CAD events was running at a higher rate among men in the thiazide group than it was among controls. Also at that time the incidence of ventricular ectopic arrhythmias in men treated with bendrofluazide had been found at a significantly higher rate than in controls.

These two observations tended to confirm earlier work linking thiazide treatment with cardiac arrhythmias (14,15) and led to two specially mounted substudies within the MRC trial (16,17). One of these showed that those receiving long-term bendrofluazide had an increased prevalence of ventricular ectopic beats (in 24-hr ECGs) compared with controls, and that this also was associated with a higher prevalence of complicated forms of ectopic beats (16). By the end of the trial, sequential analysis indicated that the excess of CAD events in men taking bendrofluazide had not increased further, and therefore it never reached significance at the 1% level, which might have led to a change in the trial protocol. However, by the end of the trial it was noted that the rate for sudden coronary deaths (occurring within 1 hr of the onset of symptoms) was significantly

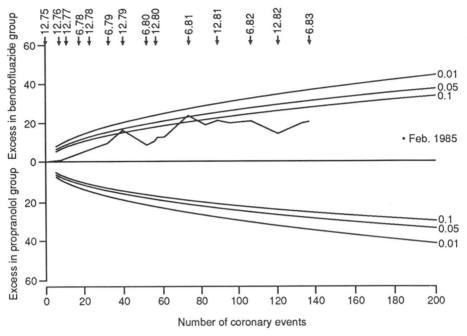

FIG. 2. MRC treatment trial for mild hypertension. Sequential chart for coronary events (men); bendrofluazide vs. propranolol. From ref. 4.

higher in men taking thiazide than it was in those taking β-blockers (Table 4). Again the incidence was higher in the thiazide and lower in the β-blocker group than it was in untreated controls; however, neither of these differences was statistically significant.

ANTIHYPERTENSIVE TREATMENT AND ECG ABNORMALITIES

ECG evidence tended to confirm the above-mentioned findings. The incidence of ECG changes suggesting transmural infarction (abnormal Q/QS items) differed between the thiazide and the β-blocker groups ($p = 0.0002$), the rate in the thiazide group being significantly higher and that in the β-blocker group being significantly lower than it was in untreated controls (Table 5). Repolarization abnormalities (ST depression with T-wave inversion) followed the same pattern in women but not in men, with higher rates in the thiazide group and lower rates in the β-blocker group than in the controls and a significant difference between the two active drug groups ($p < 0.001$). This difference was reduced but not abolished by correcting for hypokalemia (4).

Three of the earlier mild hypertension trials had undertaken analyses to determine the relationship between ECG abnormalities and the outcome of anti-

TABLE 4. *Sudden coronary deaths, and rates/1,000 person-years of observation, according to age, sex, and randomized treatment regimens*

Sex	Age	Treated				Controls	
		Bendrofluazide		Propranolol		Placebo	
		N	Rate	N	Rate	N	Rate
Male	35–44	4	1.6	1	0.4	3	0.6
	45–54	12	2.5	5	1.0	12	1.3
	55–64	13	3.6	6	1.6	26	3.5
	Total[a]	29	2.7[c]	12	1.1	41	1.9
Female	35–44	—	0.0	1	0.6	—	0.0
	45–54	2	0.5	2	0.5	1	0.1
	55–64	2	0.4	1	0.2	3	0.3
	Total[a]	4	0.4	4	0.4	4	0.2
Both	Total[a]	33	1.6[b]	16	0.7	45	1.1

From ref. 4.
Note: Rate differs significantly from propranolol group rate.
[a] Age-adjusted rates.
[b] $p < 0.05$.
[c] $p = 0.01$.

hypertensive treatment. In the MRFIT study it was found that special intervention (i.e., more active treatment) was more effective in reducing CAD mortality in nonhypertensive than it was in hypertensive men, as well as in those without rather than in those with baseline ECG abnormalities (10). A possible explanation was that some aspect of the intervention among hypertensives was having a deleterious effect, and diuretic therapy was suspected. The HDFP attempted to replicate these findings, using similar criteria to those adopted by

TABLE 5. *The incidence of ECG changes compatible with transmural infarction (Minnesota Code 1₁₋₃) according to age, sex, and randomized treatment regimens (rates/1,000 person-years of observation)*

Sex	Age	Bendrofluazide		Propranolol		Placebo	
		N	Rate	N	Rate	N	Rate
Male	35–44	28	15.5	21	11.0	40	10.6
	45–54	83	23.5	67	18.4	139	19.7
	55–64	75	28.0	61	21.6	132	23.8
	Total[a]	186	23.2*†	149	17.8	311	19.0
Female	35–44	22	19.0	8	6.6	35	15.5
	45–54	75	24.7	44	13.9	126	20.6
	55–64	70	21.0	70	20.4	154	22.7
	Total[a]	167	22.2††	122	15.7**	315	20.8
Both	Total[a]	353	22.7*†††	271	16.8*	626	19.8

From ref. 4.
Rate differs significantly from control group: ** $p < 0.01$; * $p < 0.05$.
Rate differs significantly from propranolol group: ††† $p < 0.001$; †† $p < 0.01$; † $p < 0.05$.
[a] Age-adjusted rates.

TABLE 6. *U.S. hypertension detection and follow-up program*[a]

	Stepped care		Referred care	
	No.	Rate	No.	Rate
Without ECG abnormalities				
All cardiovascular	11	14.2	12	16.1
Coronary	8	10.3	11	14.8
With ECG abnormalities				
All cardiovascular	14	44.7	12	37.7
Coronary	11	35.1	7	22.0

Note: All cardiovascular and coronary mortality according to randomized treatment and ECG status at entry. Subjects were white males.
  [a] Stratum 1.

MRFIT, and found reduced mortality in the more intensively treated stepped-care group only among those without baseline ECG abnormalities (18). Among white men with ECG abnormalities, cardiovascular and, particularly, coronary mortality was adverse in the intensively treated group (Table 6). These differences, however, were not significant, and the HDFP concluded that their findings offered no support to the MRFIT hypothesis.

A subsequent analysis of the MRFIT data (19) reported a significant interaction between ECG abnormalities and diuretic therapy in the special intervention group, with the risk of CAD death for men who were prescribed diuretics relative to men who were not prescribed diuretics estimated at 3.34 in those with ECG changes and at 0.95 in men without such changes. The most convincing evidence concerned sudden death (Table 7). An analysis of the Oslo trial data (20), using the MRFIT criteria, produced similar trends but was based on small numbers.

CIGARETTE SMOKING, ANTIHYPERTENSIVE THERAPY, AND CAD

In the MRC trial, neither the thiazide nor the β-blocker reduced CAD incidence among smokers. In male nonsmokers, CAD events were 33% less fre-

TABLE 7. *U.S. multiple risk factor intervention trial*

	Special intervention		Usual care	
	No.	Rate	No.	Rate
Without ECG abnormality				
All coronary deaths	44	15.8	58	20.7
Sudden deaths within 1 hr	19	6.8	23	8.2
With ECG abnormality				
All coronary deaths	36	29.2	21	17.7
Sudden deaths within 1 hr	21	17.0	8	6.8

Note: Coronary deaths (and rates/1000) among hypertensive men, according to randomized treatment and ECG status at entry.

quent in those treated with propranolol than among controls ($p < 0.05$) and 30% less frequent than in those receiving bendrofluazide. A similar relationship between smoking and β-blocker therapy was found in the IPPPSH trial (12). Both studies had used nonselective β-blockers, and there are pharmacological reasons that may explain why these nonselective β-blockers show benefit only in nonsmokers (21). The HAPPHY trial showed no greater CAD benefit in nonsmokers than it did in smokers treated with selective β-blockers, but it also showed no significant differences between the results of treatment with thiazides and β-blockers in any major end point. Without an untreated control group, it is difficult to determine the extent of benefit (if any) provided by either drug regimen in the HAPPHY study.

DISCUSSION

None of the recent trials, including the MRC trial, produced unequivocal evidence of CAD benefit or harm as a result of antihypertensive therapy. From the pooled data, which included all strata of HDFP, MRFIT, and EWPHE results and therefore was not restricted to mild hypertension, MacMahon and his colleagues (1) estimate an overall nonsignificant 8% reduction in CAD morbidity and mortality, compatible with an effect ranging from 18% benefit to 4% harm. This has to be contrasted with the highly significant 39% overall reduction in stroke events in the same trials.

Further work is needed to establish the apparent differences in the effects of thiazide and β-blocker treatment on stroke and CAD. In the MRC trial, both bendrofluazide and propranolol were associated with reduced stroke rates but only 18 strokes occurred in the thiazide group compared with 42 in the propranolol group, and this difference was also highly significant ($p = 0.002$); it was partly, but not entirely, attributable to better blood pressure control in the thiazide group. This unexpected and interesting difference between the two classes of drugs was not found in either the HAPPHY or IPPPSH trials. This difference remains unexplained.

CONCLUSIONS

The trials have generated a number of hypotheses concerning subgroups of hypertensive patients who may derive greater or lesser benefit from treatment. The avoidance of thiazides in men at high risk of coronary complications, and the more widespread use of β-blockers for nonsmoking men would, on present evidence, seem likely to merit further investigation; but the elimination of cigarette smoking probably would have a greater impact on CAD incidence than would any other pharmacological alternative currently available.

REFERENCES

1. MacMahon SW, Cutler JA, Furberg CD, Payne GH. The effects of treatment on morbidity and mortality from cardiovascular disease: a review of randomised controlled trials. *Prog Cardiovasc Dis* 1986;29(Suppl 1):99–118.
2. Medical Research Council Working Party on Mild to Moderate Hypertension. MRC trial of treatment of mild hypertension: principal results. *Br Med J* 1985;291:97–104.
3. Medical Research Council Working Party on Mild Hypertension. Coronary heart disease in the Medical Research Council trial of treatment of mild hypertension. *Br Heart J* 1988;59:364–378.
4. Miall WE, Greenberg G. *Mild Hypertension; Is there pressure to treat?* Cambridge: Cambridge University Press. 1987.
5. Veterans Administration Cooperative Study Group. Effects of treatment on morbidity in hypertension. Results in patients with diastolic pressure averaging 90 through 114 mm Hg. *JAMA* 1970;213:1143–1152.
6. McFate Smith W. US Public Health Service Hospitals Cooperative Study Group: treatment of mild hypertension; results of a ten-year intervention trial. *Circ Res* 1977;40(suppl):98–105.
7. Australian National Blood Pressure Study Management Committee. The Australian therapeutic trial in mild hypertension. *Lancet* 1980;1:1261–1267.
8. Helgeland A. Treatment of mild hypertension: a 5-year controlled drug trial; the Oslo study. *Am J Med* 1980;69:725–732.
9. Hypertension Detection and Follow-up Program Cooperative Research Group. Five year findings of the hypertension detection and follow-up program, (1) Reduction in mortality of persons with high blood pressure, including mild hypertension. (2) Mortality by race, sex and age. *JAMA* 1979;242:2562–2577.
10. Multiple Risk Factor Intervention Trial Research Group. Multiple Risk Factor Intervention Trial. Risk Factor changes and mortality results. *JAMA* 1982;248:1465–1477.
11. Wilhelmsen L, Berglund G, Elmfeldt D, et al. Beta-blockers versus diuretics in hypertensive men: main results from the HAPPHY trial. *J Hypertens* 1987;5:561–572.
12. IPPPSH Collaboration Group. Cardiovascular risk and risk factors in a randomised controlled trial of treatment based on a beta-blocker Oxprenolol; the International Prospective Primary Prevention Study in Hypertension. *J Hypertens* 1985;3:379–392.
13. Amery A, Birkenhager W, Brixko P, et al. Mortality and morbidity results from the European Working Party on High Blood Pressure in the Elderly Trial. *Lancet* 1985;1:1349–1354.
14. Hollifield JW, Slaton PE. Cardiac arrhythmias associated with diuretic-induced hypokalaemia and hypomagnesaemia. *Royal Society of Medicine International Congress and Symposium Series,* 1980;44:17–26.
15. Holland OB, Nixon JV, Kuthnert L. Diuretic-induced ventricular ectopic activity. *Am J Med* 1981;70:762–768.
16. Medical Research Council Working Party on Mild to Moderate Hypertension. Ventricular extrasystoles during thiazide treatment: sub-study of the MRC mild hypertension trial. *Br Med J* 1983;287:1249–1453.
17. Medical Research Council Working Party on Mild to Moderate Hypertension. Comparison of the antihypertensive efficacy and adverse reactions to two doses of bendrofluazide and hydrochlorothiazide, and the effect of potassium supplementation on the hypertensive action of bendrofluazide. *J Clin Pharmacol* 1987;27:271–277.
18. Hypertension Detection and Follow-up Program Cooperative Research Group. The effect of antihypertensive drug treatment on mortality in the presence of resting electrocardiographic abnormalities at baseline; the HDFP experience. *Circulation* 1984;70:996–1003.
19. Multiple Risk Factor Intervention Trial Research Group. Baseline rest electrocardiographic abnormalities, antihypertensive treatment, and mortality in MRFIT. *Am J Cardiol* 1985;55:1–15.
20. Holme I, Helgeland A, Hjermann I, Leren P, Lund-Larsen PG. Treatment of mild hypertension with diuretics. The importance of ECG abnormalities in the Oslo Study and in MRFIT. *JAMA* 1984;251:1298–1299.
21. Trap-Jensen J, Carlsen JE, Lysbo-Svendsen T, Christensen NJ. Cardiovascular and adrenergic effects of cigarette smoking during immediate non-selective and selective-adrenoceptor blockage in humans. *Eur J Clin Invest* 1979;9:181–183.

Atherosclerosis Reviews, Volume 21,
edited by A. Leaf and P. C. Weber.
Raven Press, Ltd., New York © 1990.

Meta-Analyses of Trials of Aspirin in Cardiovascular Disease

Julie E. Buring and Charles H. Hennekens

Departments of Medicine and Preventive Medicine, Brigham and Women's Hospital, Harvard Medical School, Brookline, Massachusetts 02146

The ability of low-dose aspirin to inhibit platelet aggregability provides a mechanism to explain its hypothesized effect in reducing risks of various manifestations of cardiovascular disease. Even at lower daily doses, which produce fewer side effects, aspirin irreversibly inhibits cyclooxygenase-dependent platelet aggregation (1).

Most (2–3), but not all (4), observational epidemiologic studies have suggested that aspirin may reduce cardiovascular disease risks by roughly 20%. As cardiovascular disease is the leading cause of morbidity and mortality in most developed countries, even such a small to moderate benefit from aspirin could have an important clinical and large public health impact. However, the amount of uncontrolled confounding in all such observational studies may be easily as large as the magnitude of the most plausible benefit. For this reason, a randomized trial of sufficiently large sample size, which distributes both known and unknown confounding variables equally between the treatment groups, is the only design strategy that can assess reliably the possible benefits of aspirin on various manifestations of cardiovascular disease.

Although a large number of randomized trials have been conducted among patients with prior cardiovascular disease, most were of small sample size and, therefore had insufficient statistical power to provide informative results. For example, 22 of the 25 trials that had been completed by 1988 were compatible with a benefit of aspirin on myocardial infarction (MI), but none achieved statistical significance. In such circumstances, an overview, or meta-analysis, which pools the data from individual trials, can provide more statistically stable estimates of the effect of aspirin on various cardiovascular disease outcomes. In an overview, the weight assigned to each trial is proportional to the number of end points, so that the results of larger trials, which include more subjects, contribute more information.

SECONDARY PREVENTION TRIALS

Secondary prevention trials of antiplatelet therapy have been conducted among patients with a history of MI, stroke, transient cerebral ischemia, and unstable angina pectoris. These trials tested aspirin, dipyridamole, or sulfinpyrazone, either alone or in combination. The 25 trials that had been completed by 1988 included over 29,000 subjects (Table 1) (5). Ten had been conducted among approximately 18,000 individuals with a prior MI, 13 involved about 9,000 patients with a history of stroke or transient cerebral ischemia, and two tested aspirin among some 2,000 subjects with unstable angina.

The three main end points analyzed were nonfatal MI, nonfatal stroke, and vascular death. In addition, to provide an overall assessment, we evaluated all important vascular events, which combined nonfatal MI, nonfatal stroke, and all vascular deaths. For subsequent nonfatal MI, the overview demonstrated a 32% reduction. For nonfatal stroke, there was a 27% decrease in risk. For total vascular mortality, the reduction was 15%. Finally, for the combined end point of all important vascular events, the overview demonstrated a 25% decrease. All these reductions were statistically significant.

When the trials were subdivided according to patient entry criteria, the trials of survivors of MI demonstrated statistically significant decreases in risk of 31% for nonfatal reinfarction, 42% for nonfatal stroke, 13% for vascular death, and 22% for any vascular event. The overview of trials of cerebrovascular disease patients (stroke and transient cerebral ischemia) demonstrated statistically significant reductions of 35% for MI, 22% for subsequent nonfatal stroke, 15% for vascular death, and 22% for any vascular event. Finally, for those entering with unstable angina, there were statistically significant decreases of 35% in nonfatal MI, 37% in vascular death, and 36% in any vascular event. The trials of unstable angina yielded too few strokes to provide meaningful data.

Thus, the overview demonstrated clear benefits of antiplatelet therapy on risks of nonfatal MI, nonfatal stroke, and vascular death among individuals

TABLE 1. *Overview of 25 trials of antiplatelet therapy in the secondary prevention of cardiovascular disease*

End point	All (25 trials)	Prior disease (entry criterion) reduction (% ± SD)		
		Cerebrovascular (13 trials)	MI (10 trials)	Unstable angina (2 trials)
Nonfatal MI	32 ± 5	35 ± 12	31 ± 5	35 ± 17
Nonfatal stroke	27 ± 6	22 ± 7	42 ± 11	—
Total cardiovascular death	15 ± 4	15 ± 7	13 ± 5	37 ± 19
Any vascular event	25 ± 3	22 ± 5	22 ± 4	36 ± 13

TABLE 2. *Direct and indirect comparisons between various antiplatelet therapies from the overview for important vascular events*

Indirect comparisons	Difference in favor of antiplatelet therapy (% + SD)
Aspirin 0.9–1.5 g daily vs. nil	23 ± 4
Aspirin 0.3 g daily vs. nil	24 ± 8
Sulfinpyrazone vs. nil	17 ± 8
Aspirin + dipyridamole vs. nil	31 ± 5
Direct comparisons (total events/patients)	Difference in favor of aspirin (% ± SD)
Aspirin vs. sulfinpyrazone (54/346 vs. 74/357)	28 ± 17
Aspirin vs. aspirin + dipyridamole (275/1597 vs. 279/1597)	2 ± 9

with prior cardiovascular events. In addition, the overview also suggested that aspirin, which is the safest, least expensive, and most convenient form of anti-platelet therapy, is at least as effective as the other antiplatelet agents in reducing risks of cardiovascular disease (Table 2). Specifically, there was no clear evidence that aspirin plus dypridamole is any more effective than aspirin alone, because the indirect comparison between the two risk reductions is not significant, and the overview of the direct comparisons indicates no difference whatsoever.

PRIMARY PREVENTION TRIALS

Two randomized trials of aspirin in primary prevention have been completed (Table 3), both among male physicians. One, the Physicians' Health Study (6), randomized 22,071 U.S. physicians, aged 40 to 84 years, the other, the British Doctors' Trial (7), randomized 5139 U.K. doctors, aged 50 to 78 years.

The U.S. trial tested 325 mg aspirin on alternate days, utilizing a double-

TABLE 3. *Aspirin in primary prevention: U.S. Physicians' Health Study and British Doctors' Trial*

End point	Reduction (% ± SD)		
	U.S. Physicians' Health Study	British Doctors' Trial	Overview
Nonfatal MI	39 ± 9	3 ± 19	32 ± 8
Nonfatal stroke	↑19 ± 15	↑13 ± 24	↑18 ± 13
Total cardiovascular death	2 ± 15	7 ± 14	5 ± 10
Any vascular event	18 ± 7	4 ± 12	13 ± 6

↑ = Nonsignificant increased risk of stroke among aspirin-allocated subjects.

blind, placebo-controlled, 2×2 factorial design, which allowed for the independent testing of the effects of β-carotene supplementation on risks of cancer. The aspirin group experienced a 44% reduction in risk of MI compared with those assigned placebo, reflecting significant benefits on both fatal and nonfatal events. When the analysis was restricted to nonfatal MI, the reduction was 39%. For the combined end point of nonfatal MI, nonfatal stroke, and vascular death, there was a statistically significant 18% reduction in the aspirin group. The U.S. trial found an apparent 19% increase in nonfatal stroke, but this did not achieve statistical significance.

The British Doctors' Trial tested a daily dose of 500 mg aspirin, with the control group simply asked to avoid aspirin or any aspirin-containing compounds. Although participants were aware of their assignment, the investigators remained blinded to treatment assignments. In the British trial, there was no significant difference between the two groups for nonfatal MI, nonfatal stroke, vascular death, or the combined end point of any important vascular event.

There were several important differences between the two primary prevention trials. In terms of design, the U.S. trial was double-blind and placebo-controlled, whereas the British trial used a single-blind, open design. As regards dose and frequency of administration, the U.S. trial tested 325 mg on alternate days, whereas the British trial tested a daily dose of 500 mg. Finally, the most important difference between the trials was sample size, with 22,071 randomized in the U.S. trial, compared with 5,139 in the U.K. trial. Because the U.S. trial was so much larger, an overview of the U.S. and British trials (8) demonstrated a highly significant 32% reduction in risk of nonfatal MI. There was also a nonsignificant 18% apparent increase in nonfatal stroke and a nonsignificant 5% reduction in cardiovascular mortality, but the confidence intervals were very wide for both these end points. Thus, the data are not informative enough to make any meaningful inferences concerning the primary prevention of stroke and vascular death by aspirin.

CURRENT KNOWLEDGE CONCERNING ASPIRIN AND CARDIOVASCULAR DISEASE

The overview of secondary prevention trials demonstrated clear benefits of aspirin for patients with a previous MI, stroke, transient ischemic attack, or unstable angina. In such patients, aspirin produced definite reductions in the risks of subsequent MI, stroke or vascular death, and in 1985, the U.S. Food and Drug Administration (FDA) approved the prescription labeling of aspirin for treatment of patients with a prior MI or unstable angina.

With regard to the most serious potential adverse effect of antiplatelet therapy, hemorrhagic stroke, the overview did demonstrate a statistically significant decrease in total stroke, so any postulated increased risk of the rare but serious hemorrhagic stroke would be far outweighed by the protective effects of aspirin on the far more common strokes of thrombotic etiology.

Concerning primary prevention, the U.S. Physicians' Health Study has demonstrated a clear reduction in MI associated with low-dose aspirin. However, the evidence concerning stroke and vascular mortality remains inconclusive because of inadequate numbers of end points in both primary prevention trials of aspirin as well as in the overview of their results. With respect to risk of hemorrhagic stroke, the U.S. data raised the possibility of an increased risk of such events associated with aspirin. The British study reported an increase in "disabling" strokes among those assigned aspirin, but it remains unclear whether this represents an increase in hemorrhagic strokes, which are typically more severe than thrombotic events, or reflects some bias due to subjective assessment of residual disability.

With regard to the use of aspirin in primary prevention at present, prophylactic therapy seems most appropriate for those whose risk for MI is sufficiently high to warrant the adverse effects of the drug. In October 1989, The Cardiology and Renal Drugs Advisory Committee of the FDA voted to recommend that the results of the U.S. Physicians' Health Study be incorporated into the professional labeling of aspirin to reduce risks of a first MI in apparently healthy men.

As regards generalization, the U.S. male physicians were much healthier than men in the general public, and there is little reason to believe that these benefits would not extend to less healthy populations. The absolute benefits, in fact, would be greater in higher-risk populations, because the absolute risks of cardiovascular disease are so much higher. As regards aspirin prophylaxis in women, there is no direct evidence on this question. It may be prudent, however, to assume that women at sufficiently high risk for MI also would benefit from aspirin. Of course, it would be optimal to test this question directly in a large-scale randomized trial of women.

It is important to view the benefits of aspirin in primary prevention of MI in the context of what is known already about modification of other cardiovascular risk factors. For example, with regard to blood cholesterol, a 10% decrease corresponds to a roughly 20% to 30% reduction in risks of cardiovascular disease (9). For blood pressure, a 6 mm decrease in diastolic pressure among those with mild to moderate hypertension appears to lower risks of coronary heart disease by 12% and stroke by about 40% (10). Finally, cessation of cigarette smoking results in an approximately 50% decrease in coronary heart disease, perhaps even within a matter of months (11).

Thus, the prescription of aspirin should be viewed as an adjunct, not alternative, to control or elimination of other cardiovascular risk factors. In addition, aspirin should be initiated only on the recommendation of a physician or other primary health care provider. Such an individual judgment should consider the cardiovascular risk profile of the patient, the known side effects of aspirin, and these newly documented benefits on various manifestations of cardiovascular disease in different categories of individuals (7).

REFERENCES

1. Moncada S, Vane JR. Arachidonic acid metabolites and the interactions between platelets and blood-vessel walls. *N Engl J Med* 1979;300:1142–1147.
2. Hennekens CH, Karlson LA, Rosner B. A case-control study of regular aspirin use and coronary heart deaths. *Circulation* 1978;58:35–38.
3. Hammond EC, Garfinkel L. Aspirin and coronary heart disease: findings of a prospective study. *Br Med J* 1975;2:269.
4. Paganini-Hill A, Chao A, Ross RK, Henderson BE. Aspirin use and chronic diseases: a cohort study of the elderly. *Br Med J* 1989;299:1247–1250.
5. Anti-Platelet Trialists' Collaboration. Secondary prevention of vascular disease by prolonged anti-platelet therapy. *Br Med J* 1988;296:320–332.
6. Steering Committee of the Physicians' Health Study Research Group. Final report on the aspirin component of the ongoing Physicians' Health Study. *N Eng J Med* 1989;321:129–135.
7. Peto R, Gray R, Collins R, et al. A randomised trial of the effects of prophylactic daily aspirin among male British doctors. *Br Med J* 1988;296:313–316.
8. Hennekens CH, Buring JE, Sandercock P, Collins R, Peto R. Aspirin and other antiplatelet agents in the secondary and primary prevention of cardiovascular disease. *Circulation* 1989;80: 749–756.
9. Peto R, Yusuf S, Collins R. Cholesterol-lowering trial results in their epidemiologic context. *Circulation* 1985;72(Suppl 3):451.
10. Hebert PR, Fiebach NH, Eberlein KA, Taylor JO, Hennekens CH. The community-based randomized trials of pharmacologic treatment of mild-to-moderate hypertension. *Am J Epidemiol* 1988;127:581–590.
11. Hennekens CH, Buring JE, Mayrent S. Smoking, aging and coronary heart disease. In: Bosse R, ed. *Smoking and Aging,* Lexington, MA: D. C. Heath, 1984:95–115.

Atherosclerosis Reviews, Volume 21,
edited by A. Leaf and P. C. Weber.
Raven Press, Ltd., New York © 1990.

Atherosclerosis Regression in Humans

David H. Blankenhorn

Department of Medicine, Atherosclerosis Research Institute, University of Southern California School of Medicine, Los Angeles, California 90033

In 1924, as a result of his observations on the effects of a marked decrease in dietary fat during World War I, Aschoff (1) inferred that regression of human atherosclerosis might be possible. After World War II, Malmros (2) and Strom and Jensen (3) related dietary restrictions of eggs and butter to temporarily reduced ischemic heart disease (IHD) mortality rates in Scandinavia. Similar observations were made in Leningrad, Russia, where there was an apparent decrease in myocardial infarction during the siege, and a reappearance of manifest coronary disease when food supplies were restored (4). Schettler (5) reviewed autopsy findings during three postwar periods and associated progressive decreases in numbers of atherosclerotic lesions seen at post postmorten with war-related, severe dietary deprivation. Wilens (6) found smaller and less severe lesions in patients who had suffered more drastic weight losses prior to death. He concluded that lipids were being withdrawn from arterial deposits in relatively short periods of time among those patients who had lost from 15 to 110 lbs within 1 year before autopsy. Other observations of atherosclerotic improvement associated with wasting disease have been described in studies of anorexia nervosa (7) and carcinoma (8 11).

FIRST ANGIOGRAPHIC STUDIES

The earliest report of atherosclerotic improvement was from Scandinavia. Three patients among 31 reported by Ost and Stenson treated with 3 to 6 g of nicotinic acid showed improvement in femoral angiograms after 3 years. Angiographic change was accompanied by an increase in pulse volume and improved walking capacity (12). Lipid levels achieved by niacin therapy were not reported, but this dose of niacin is known to produce major reductions in low-density lipoprotein (LDL) cholesterol and concomitant increases in high-density lipoprotein (HDL) cholesterol.

DePalma reported a 57-year-old diabetic who reduced his serum cholesterol from 327 to 190 mg%, quit smoking, and began an exercise program. Serial angiograms showed the disappearance of a popliteal-obstructing lesion after 9 months (13). Three among eight patients treated by Thompson with plasma exchange showed measurable improvement (14). Roth and Kostuk reported a 56-year-old man with episodic dyspnea, angina, and a single left anterior descending coronary lesion on arteriography (15). With self-imposed diet modification and increased exercise, his serum cholesterol was reduced from 269 to 201 mg and triglycerides from 205 to 93 mg%. After 1 year, angiography revealed decreased stenosis in the left anterior descending lesion accompanied by increased myocardial perfusion by thallium scanning.

The first report from our laboratory was a study of 25 hyperlipidemic patients treated with diet, lipid-lowering medication (primarily clofibrate and neomycin) and antihypertensive medication, if indicated. Nine patients showed regression in femoral atherosclerosis after 13 months (16). Patients showing regression were those with a significant reduction in blood total cholesterol (from 311 to 246 mg%), triglyceride (from 362 to 143 mg%), systolic (from 132 to 123 mm Hg) and diastolic (from 85 to 79 mm Hg) blood pressure levels. Patients showing progression did not have significant reduction in these risk factors.

Kuo reported that treatment with combined colestipol and niacin therapy could stabilize atherosclerotic coronary lesions for periods as long as $7\frac{1}{2}$ years. This evidence was based on serial coronary angiographic examinations (17). In 1984, Malinow tabulated cases in the literature showing angiographic evidence of regression and found over 100 such cases (18).

THE FIRST CONTROLLED CLINICAL TRIALS

Duffield and co-workers (19) conducted an open, randomized study of advanced femoral atherosclerosis where patients were treated with lipid-lowering drugs assigned according to their Fredrickson phenotype. Entry criteria were claudication of 6 months' duration and plasma cholesterol levels over 250 mg%. Patients with diabetes, diastolic hypertension, and rest pain were excluded. There were 12 drug-treated subjects whose average age was 55 years and 12 "usual care" patients whose average age was matched and whose lipids were untreated. Type II patients were treated with 12 to 24 g of cholestyramine a day plus 3 to 6 g of niacin. Type IV patients were treated with niacin; Type III patients were treated with clofibrate. Angiograms were repeated after 13 months. Ten among 144 segments in treated patients showed lesion progression; 27 among 156 segments in the usual care showed progression. This difference was significant at the 0.01 level, demonstrating an effect in retarding the process of atherosclerosis progression. The number of subjects was too small to analyze by trial on a per patient basis.

The National Heart, Lung and Blood Institute Type II Study was a randomized, placebo-controlled and double-blind study (20). It tested the effects of 24 g of cholestyramine with coronary angiography in subjects with Type II hyperlipoproteinemia and overt coronary disease. Average entry levels were: total cholesterol, 323 mg/dl; triglyceride, 164 mg/dl; HDL cholesterol, 39 mg/dl; and

LDL cholesterol, 251 mg/dl. The drug and placebo groups were evenly matched. A low-fat diet reduced LDL cholesterol levels by 5% in both groups. During the interval between angiograms, LDL cholesterol levels in the placebo group were reduced an additional 5% and LDL cholesterol levels in the cholestyramine group were reduced by 26%.

The original study design called for 250 patients randomized to two treatment arms, but recruitment was stopped after 54 months when 143 patients had been randomized. Eventually, 116 subjects (57 placebo, 59 cholestyramine) had second angiograms and these were evaluated in pairs with the temporal sequence and treatment masked. Subjects were classified as definite progression, probable progression, definite regression, probable regression, mixed response, and no change. Definite progression was found in 35% of placebo- versus 25% of drug-treated subjects, probable progression in 14% placebo- versus 7% drug-treated subjects, no change in 42% of placebo- versus 53% of drug-treated subjects, and probable regression in 5% of placebo- versus 3% of drug-treated subjects. Definite regression was found in 2% of placebo- versus 3% of drug-treated subjects. A mixed response with lesions changing in opposite directions in the same subject was found in 2% of placebo- and 8% of drug-treated subjects. The overall conclusion of the investigators was that although, the number of subjects evaluated did not allow definite conclusions, the outcome suggested that cholestyramine retarded the progression of coronary atherosclerosis. An additional conclusion drawn after baseline demographic inequalities and lesion severity were taken into account was that a treatment effect in retarding progression could be demonstrated in a group of lesions with $\geq 50\%$ stenosis because 33% of placebo- versus 12% of cholestyramine-treated lesions of this sort showed progression ($p < 0.05$).

The Leiden Intervention Trial, which began in 1978 and ended in 1981, presented evidence of a diet effect on coronary atherosclerosis (21). Sixty-one patients with stable angina, one or more lesions exceeding 50% stenosis, and who were not candidates for coronary bypass surgery were recruited. The trial was not randomized or blinded; however, coronary angiograms were evaluated by readers who did not know blood lipid levels or the order of examination. All patients were assigned to a vegetarian diet, which reduced saturated fat and cholesterol while it increased polyunsaturated fat. It was estimated that the diet at entry provided 11% of calories from saturated fat and 8.5% from unsaturated fat and that daily cholesterol intake was 88 mg/1,000 calories. After 1 year, diet estimates indicated 6.6% of calories came from saturated fat, 16.8% came from polyunsaturated fat, and daily cholesterol intake was 30 mg/1,000 calories. Among 53 who started the diet, four died in the first year (three with myocardial infarction; one suddenly) and seven patients had coronary artery bypass grafting. Repeat angiography was not performed in three patients (because of a malignant tumor in two and refusal in one). Thirty-nine patients were restudied and films were evaluated both by visual inspection and computer analysis (21). Twenty-one among 39 patients showed progression and 18 showed no progression. Among those without progression, total cholesterol reduction was 23 mg%.

CONTROLLED TRIALS SHOWING REGRESSION

The Cholesterol Lowering Atherosclerosis Study (CLAS I) was a selectively blinded, placebo-controlled trial with end points in native coronary arteries, aortocoronary venous bypass grafts, and femoral and carotid arteries (22). One hundred eighty-eight subjects were randomized to one of two treatment arms; drug plus diet or placebo plus diet. Subjects were nonsmoking men aged 40 to 59 years with previous coronary bypass surgery. Total plasma cholesterol levels at entry ranged from 185 to 350 mg%. Combined colestipol plus niacin therapy produced 26% reduction in total plasma cholesterol levels, 43% reduction in LDL cholesterol levels, and 22% reduction in plasma triglyceride levels, plus simultaneous 37% elevation of HDL cholesterol levels. One hundred sixty-two subjects had completed 2 years of combined treatment with colestipol at the time the study was truncated because coronary angiograms demonstrated clear benefits from therapy. Coronary angiograms were reviewed by a panel of expert angiographers as a safety surveillance measure prior to assessment by computerized image processing (23).

Treatment produced a significant reduction in progression of atherosclerosis in native coronary arteries, both in the average number of lesions that progressed per subject ($p < 0.03$) and in the percent of subjects with new atheroma formation ($p < 0.03$). The average number of native coronary lesions in drug-treated subjects was 10.9 per subject and the average number showing increased stenosis was 1 per subject. The average number of native coronary lesions in placebo-treated subjects was 11.2 per subject and the average number showing increased stenosis was 1.4 per subject. Among 80 drug-treated subjects, 8 (10%) developed new native coronary lesions, among 82 placebo-treated subjects, 18 (22%) developed new native coronary lesions.

In bypass grafts, treatment also significantly reduced the percent of subjects with any adverse change ($p < 0.03$) and percent of subjects with new lesions ($p < 0.04$). The average number of grafts in both drug-treated and placebo subjects was 2.7. Among drug-treated subjects, 24% showed an adverse change (increased stenosis or increased diffuse edge irregularity) in one or more bypass grafts, among placebo subjects 39% showed an adverse change in bypass grafts. Fourteen (18%) among 80 drug-treated subjects developed new graft lesions, 25 (30%) among 82 placebo-treated subjects developed new graft lesions.

The deterioration observed in overall status of the coronary arteries as judged from the extent of obstructive lesions in native coronary arteries and/or abnormalities of bypass grafts was significantly less in drug-treated subjects than it was in placebo-treated subjects ($p < 0.001$). In fact, evidence of atherosclerosis regression, as indicated by perceptible improvement in overall coronary status, occurred in 16.2% of colestipol-niacin-treated subjects versus 3.6% of placebo-treated subjects, ($p = 0.007$). Evidence for benefit retained strong statistical significance after CLAS results were divided to compare treatment effects separately when entry cholesterol levels were above or below 240 mg/dl.

CLAS II was an optional extension of CLAS I in which study subjects stayed on their assigned medication, either drug or placebo, for another 2 years and had a third angiogram. One hundred three subjects (56 drug, 47 placebo) had completed CLAS II before the last subject to enter CLAS I had completed a final CLAS I angiogram and the beneficial effects of therapy became known. A recent analysis of the experience of these 103 subjects over 4 years indicates that the lipid changes were well maintained and that the therapy effect seen at 2 years was strongly evident at 4 years. The global change score that demonstrated significant benefit at 2 years ($p < 0.007$) showed further divergence between drug and placebo at 4 years ($p < 0.001$). At 4 years, perceptible regression was seen in overall coronary status in 17.9% of subjects in the drug group and in 6.4% of the placebo group (24).

A three-arm trial comparing conventional therapy with colestipol (30 g/day) plus niacin (4 g/day) or colestipol (30 g/day) plus lovastatin (40 mg/day) was reported in November 1989 (25). Subjects were men under 62 years of age with proven coronary artery disease and apolipoprotein B levels > 125 mg%. LDL Cholesterol levels were reduced 34% by colestipol plus niacin and 48% by colestipol plus lovastatin. HDL Cholesterol levels were increased 41% by colestipol plus niacin and 14% by colestipol plus lovastatin. Coronary angiograms were hand-traced and the tracings were digitized for further analysis. Subjects were classified as showing regression or progression on the basis of average change in nine standardized proximal segments and significant benefits ($p < 0.006$) were demonstrated for both treatment arms as compared to conventional therapy.

A smaller two-arm trial in progress is testing rigorous fat dietary restriction, stress reduction, and modification of lifestyle in 48 subjects. An encouraging interim report describes changes in 142 lesions in 29 subjects who have completed two angiograms (26).

REDUCTION OF NEW LESION FORMATION

An unexpected bonus from studies of regression has been information on the formation of new coronary lesions. Formation of new lesions in both native coronary arteries and aortocoronary bypass grafts was found after 2 years of colestipol plus niacin therapy in CLAS and confirmed again at 4 years. In patients with established coronary artery disease, these findings have obvious implications for primary prevention of ischemic heart disease and offer promise for eventual successful control of the atherosclerosis and its complications.

SUMMARY

Evidence that human atherosclerosis is a reversible condition has been accumulating for more than half a century. The first indications were from starved populations and patients with wasting disease. More direct evidence became available when serial angiograms were used to follow the course of patients treated to reduce atherosclerotic risk factors. The earliest controlled clinical trials employing angiography with relatively smaller numbers of subjects and a moderate lowering of blood lipid level demonstrated that lesion progression could be reduced. Later trials with more subjects and/or a more aggressive reduction of blood lipid level have demonstrated regression. There is additional evidence that dietary change can reduce progression and preliminary reports of regression with rigid dietary fat restriction. An important bonus from the studies of human atherosclerotic lesions is evidence that the rate of formation of new coronary lesions can be reduced.

REFERENCES

1. Aschoff L. *Lectures in Pathology.* New York: Hoeber, 1924.
2. Malmros H. The relation of nutrition to health. A statistical study of the effect of the wartime on arteriosclerosis, cardiosclerosis, tuberculosis and diabetes. *Acta Med Scand* [*suppl*] 1950;246:137–150.
3. Strom A, Jensen RA. Mortality from circulatory diseases in Norway 1940–1945. *Lancet* 1951;1: 126.
4. Brozek J, Wells S, Keys A. Medical aspects of semistarvation and Leningrad (seige 1941–42). *Am Rev Soviet Med* 1946;4:70.
5. Schettler G. Cardiovascular diseases during and after World War II: a comparison of the Federal Republic of Germany with other European countries. *Prev Med* 1979;8:581.
6. Wilens SL. The resorption of arterial atheromatous deposits in wasting disease. *Am J Pathol* 1947;23:793.
7. Mordasini R, Klose G, Greten H. Secondary type II hyperlipoproteinemia in patients with anorexia nervosa. *Metabolism* 1978;27:71.
8. London JW, Rosenberg SE, Draper JW, Almy TP. The effect of estrogens on atherosclerosis. *Am J Int Med* 1961;55:63.
9. Rivin AU, Dimitroff SP. The incidence and severity of atherosclerosis in estrogen-treated males and in females with hypoestrogenic or a hyperestrogenic state. *Circulation* 1954;9:533.
10. McGill HC. Fatty streaks in the coronary arteries and aorta. *Lab Invest* 1968;18:560.
11. Berry JF, Resch JA, Baker AB. Serum lipids and cerebral atherosclerosis in terminal cancer patients. *Neurology* 1966;16:673.
12. Ost RC, Stenson S. Regression of peripheral atherosclerosis during therapy with high doses of nicotinic acid. *Scand J Clin Lab Invest* [*suppl*] 1967;99:241–245.
13. DePalma RG, Hubay CA, Insull W Jr, Robinson AV, Hartman PH. Progression and regression of experimental atherosclerosis. *Surg Gynecol Obstet* 1970;131:633–647.
14. Thompson GR, Lowenthal R, Myant MD. Plasma exchange in management of homozygous familial hypercholesterolemia. *Lancet* 1975;1:1208.
15. Roth D, Kostuk WJ. Noninvasive and invasive demonstration of spontaneous regression of coronary artery disease. *Circulation* 1980;62:888–896.
16. Barndt R Jr, Blankenhorn DH, Crawford DW. Regression and progression of early femoral atherosclerosis in treated hyperlipoproteinemic patients. *Ann Intern Med* 1977;86:139–146.
17. Kuo PT, Hayase K, Kostis JB, Moreyra AE. Use of combined diet and colestipol in long-term (7–$7\frac{1}{2}$ years) treatment of patients with type II hyperlipoproteinemia. *Circulation* 1979;59:199–211.

18. Malinow MR. Atherosclerosis: progression, regression, and resolution. *Am Heart J* 1984;108: 1523–1537.
19. Duffield RG, Lewis B, Miller NE, Jamieson CW, Brunt JN, Colchester AC. Treatment of hyperlipidaemia retards progression of symptomatic femoral atherosclerosis. A randomised controlled trial. *Lancet* 1983;2:639–642.
20. Brensike JF, Levy RI, Kelsey SF, et al. Effects of therapy with cholestyramine on progression of coronary arteriosclerosis: results of the NHLBI Type II Coronary Intervention Study. *Circulation* 1984;69:313–324.
21. Arntzenius AC, Kromhout D, Barth JD, et al. Diet, lipoproteins, and the progression of coronary atherosclerosis. The Leiden Intervention Trial. *N Engl J Med* 1985;312:805–811.
22. Blankenhorn DH, Nessim SA, Johnson RL, Sanmarco ME, Azen SP, Cashin-Hemphill L. Beneficial effects of combined colestipol-niacin therapy on coronary atherosclerosis and coronary venous bypass grafts. *JAMA* 1987;257:3233–3240.
23. Blankenhorn DH, Johnson RL, Nessim SA, Azen SP, Sanmarco ME, Selzer RH. The Cholesterol Lowering Atherosclerosis Study (CLAS): Design, Methods, and Baseline Results. *Controlled Clin Trials* 1987;8:354–387.
24. Cashin-Hemphill L, Sanmarco ME, Blankenhorn DH. Augmented beneficial effects of Colestipol-niacin therapy at four years in the CLAS Trial [Abstract]. *Circulation* 1989;80:II-381.
25. Brown BG, Lin JT, Schaefer SM, Kaplan CA, Dodge HT, Albers JJ. Niacin or Lovastatin, combined with Colestipol, regress coronary atherosclerosis and prevent clinical events in men with elevated apolipoprotein B [Abstract]. *Circulation* 1989;80:II-266.
26. Ornish DM, Scherwitz LW, Brown SE, et al. Adherence to lifestyle changes and reversal of coronary atherosclerosis [Abstract]. *Circulation* 1989;80:II-57.
27. Lichtlen PR, Hugenholtz P, Rafflenbeul W, Jost S, Hecker H. Retardation of the progression of coronary artery disease with nifedipine. Results of INTACT [Abstract]. *Circulation* 1989;80: II-382.

Atherosclerosis Reviews, Volume 21,
edited by A. Leaf and P. C. Weber.
Raven Press, Ltd., New York © 1990.

Mechanisms of Platelet Inhibition by Prostacyclin:

New Aspects

Wolfgang Siess

Institut für Prophylaxe und Epidemiologie der Kreislaufkrankheiten, Universität München, D 8-München 2, Federal Republic of Germany

Prostacyclin (PGI_2) is the most powerful inhibitor of platelet function (1). PGI_2, prostaglandin E_1, and the stable PGI_2-analog iloprost bind to a common specific receptor on the platelet surface that couples to the guanine nucleotide-binding protein G_s, which stimulates adenylate cyclase. Incubation of platelets with these agonists leads to an increase of cyclic AMP and the cyclic AMP-dependent phosphorylation of proteins with the molecular weights 22, 24, 50, 130, and 250 kDa (2). In addition, we recently found that PGI_2 induced the phosphorylation of platelet proteins of 30, 38, and 60 kDa molecular weight (W. Siess, unpublished observations). Cyclic AMP–dependent phosphorylation of platelet proteins is most likely responsible for its inhibition of platelet function. Platelet shape change, adhesion to subendothelium, secretion, and aggregation are suppressed completely by pretreatment of platelets with PGI_2. In comparison, inhibition of platelet cyclooxygenase by aspirin has only a dampening effect on platelet aggregation; platelet shape change, adhesion, and primary aggregation are not inhibited (Table 1). In addition, aspirin has no effect on platelet secretion and aggregation induced by high doses of thrombin or collagen (2).

CYCLIC AMP INHIBITS PHOSPHOLIPASE C-ACTIVATION

Currently it is assumed that one of the main mechanisms by which an increase of cyclic AMP inhibits stimulus-induced platelet activation is the inhibition of receptor-mediated phosphoinositide hydrolysis and subsequent protein kinase C (PKC) activation and calcium mobilization. The inhibitory action of cyclic AMP on fibrinogen receptor exposure, myosin light-chain phosphorylation, actin polymerization, and cytoskeletal assembly are considered to be consequences of the inhibition of receptor-mediated phospholipase C activation. Other studies, however, have indicated that further target sites exist that are

159

TABLE 1. *Effects of cyclooxygenase inhibition by aspirin and of increases of cyclic AMP levels by prostacyclin (PGI$_2$) on platelet responses*

Platelet responses	Inhibition by	
	Aspirin	PGI$_2$
Shape change	—	+
Adhesion	—	+
Secretion	+	+
Aggregation		
Primary	—	+
Secondary	+	+

important for platelet inhibition by cyclic AMP. For example, it has been reported by several investigators that cyclic AMP inhibits secretion and aggregation induced by Ca^{2+}-ionophore at steps distal to calcium mobilization (2,3). Also, modest increments in platelet cyclic AMP have been reported to abolish platelet-activating factor–induced aggregation and secretion, but to have little effect on phosphoinositide hydrolysis and elevation of cytosolic calcium induced by platelet-activating factor (4).

Many studies indicate that phosphorylation of the 20- and 47-kDa proteins are related closely to platelet functional responses: myosin light-chain kinase (MLCK)-dependent phosphorylation of myosin light-chain may trigger shape change, whereas PKC-dependent phosphorylation of the 47 kDa polypeptide may regulate aggregation and secretion (2,5,6). Therefore, we decided to undertake a study to find out whether increasing platelet cyclic AMP could suppress aggregation by inhibiting PKC or Ca^{2+}-dependent kinases involved in the activation of platelets.

CYCLIC AMP INHIBITS PLATELET AGGREGATION AT STEPS DISTAL TO ACTIVATION OF PROTEIN KINASE C AND Ca^{2+}-DEPENDENT PROTEIN KINASE

The effect of prostacyclin on platelet activation induced by phorbol ester and Ca^{2+}-ionophore was studied (3). Phorbol ester and Ca^{2+}-ionophores activate platelets through different mechanisms and can be used specifically to probe the PKC-dependent pathway and the Ca^{2+} pathway of platelet activation, respectively (2). Phorbol esters, by intercalation into the membrane without mobilization of calcium, translocate PKC from the cytosol to the membrane and induce the PKC-dependent phosphorylation of various proteins, such as the 47-kDa polypeptide and the 20-kDa myosin light-chain (2). Ca^{2+}-ionophores activate platelets through Ca^{2+}-influx and -mobilization from intracellular stores. The increase in cytosolic Ca^{2+} leads to the activation of Ca^{2+}/calmodulin-dependent kinases, such as MLCK, which phosphorylates myosin light-

chain (20 kDa), and to a Ca^{2+}-dependent activation of PKC, which phosphorylates a 47-kDa protein.

We found that the phorbol ester, phorbol 12,13-dibutyrate, (PdBu), in the
absence of any increase of cytosolic Ca^{2+}, induced the phosphorylations of proteins with molecular masses of 20, 38, and 47 kDa. High concentrations of
phorbol 12,13-dibutyrate (>50 nM) were needed to observe a significant aggregation response. Dose-dependency and time courses of the 20-kDa myosin
light-chain phosphorylation were different from those for the 47 kDa-protein:
The phosphorylation of the 47-kDa protein occurred earlier and at lower concentrations of PdBu than did the 20-kDa protein phosphorylation. A close temporal relationship between phorbol-ester-induced 20-kDa protein phosphorylation and platelet aggregation was found, suggesting a role for PKC-dependent
myosin phosphorylation in inducing platelet aggregation. However, we found
that preincubation of platelets with PGI_2 completely suppressed aggregation
without affecting the phosphorylation of any protein evoked by phorbol ester
(3). PGI_2 stimulation of the phosphorylation of the 50-kDa protein by protein
kinase A closely correlated with the inhibition of PdBu-induced aggregation
by PGI_2. It was concluded from these data that phorbol esters induce platelet
aggregation through PKC-dependent phosphorylation of specific proteins, but
that distal to this event are steps crucial for the regulation of platelet aggregation,
which are target sites for cyclic AMP–dependent protein kinases (Fig. 1). Such
sites could be the glycoprotein IIb/IIIa complex (which represents the fibrinogen receptor) or, more likely, as yet unknown proteins that regulate the confor-
mational change and the expression of the fibrinogen receptor on platelet activation.

Ca^{2+}-ionophore A23187, at 0.1 μM, induced shape change and a pronounced
phosphorylation of the 20-kDa myosin light chain, but no or only a small phosphorylation of the 47-kDa protein. We observed that, by increasing the concentration of A23187 from 0.2 to 1 μM, aggregation and phosphorylation of the
47-kDa protein increased progressively, whereas the stimulation of the 20-kDa
myosin light-chain phosphorylation remained unchanged. These results sup-

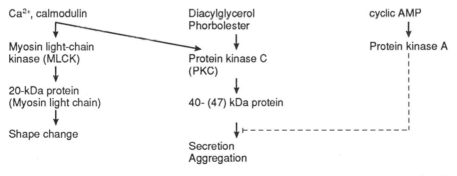

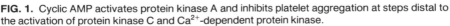

FIG. 1. Cyclic AMP activates protein kinase A and inhibits platelet aggregation at steps distal to
the activation of protein kinase C and Ca^{2+}-dependent protein kinase.

port the idea that myosin light-chain phosphorylation is related to shape change and a prerequisite for aggregation, whereas PKC-dependent phosphorylation of the 47-kDa protein is more involved in regulation of aggregation and secretion (5,6). Preincubation of platelets with PGI_2 neither inhibited Ca^{2+} mobilization, 20-kDa myosin light-chain phosphorylation and shape change, nor reduced 47-kDa protein phosphorylation, but it did inhibit platelet aggregation induced by Ca^{2+}-ionophore A23187 (3). These results indicate that cyclic AMP inhibits platelet aggregation at steps distal to Ca^{2+} mobilization and Ca^{2+}-dependent phosphorylation of 20- and 47-kDa proteins (Fig. 1), and they point again to the fibrinogen receptor and proteins interacting with the fibrinogen receptor as possible target sites for cyclic AMP–dependent protein kinases.

Rap1B, A ras-LIKE PROTEIN, IS PHOSPHORYLATED BY CYCLIC AMP–DEPENDENT PROTEIN KINASE

A further study was designed to obtain structural information of one protein that is phosphorylated by protein kinase A in platelets, the microsomal 22 kDa protein (2). Cyclic AMP–dependent phosphorylation of P22, recently named thrombolamban (7), stimulates Ca^{2+} uptake into platelet membrane vesicles (2,8). The stimulation of Ca^{2+} transport from the cytosol into the dense tubular system might explain the rapid fall in cytoplasmic Ca^{2+} that is observed when adenylate cyclase stimulators are added after the maximal platelet responses evoked by platelet stimuli (2). P22 is a major membrane protein in human platelets that is visible by Coomassie blue stain of membrane proteins separated on a SDS/polyacrylamide gel (9). P22 binds GTP on nitrocellulose blots and displays strong immunoreactivity with the monoclonal antibody, M90 (10). This antibody recognizes an epitope of the H-ras p21 protein that comprises a major GTP-binding region (amino acids 107–130). The 22 kDa phosphorylated protein was isolated from the membrane fraction of ^{32}P-labeled platelets that had been incubated with iloprost, a stable PGI_2-analog. The phosphorylated 22-kDa protein was isolated by excision of the labeled band from preparative SDS-polyacrylamide gels and subsequent electroelution of the protein from the gel. Phosphoamino acid analysis revealed that the 22-kDa protein was phosphorylated primarily at a serine residue. Enzymatic cleavage of the purified protein by trypsin and *S. aureus* V8 protease produced ^{32}P-labeled peptides, which were separated by HPLC and underwent amino acid sequence determination. The HPLC profile of the cleavage products obtained by both trypsin and V8 protease showed a major radioactive peak that eluted with a late retention time indicating that the peptide was very hydrophobic. Amino acid sequence analysis of the labeled peptides revealed that the phosphorylated P22 was identical to rap1B (9), one member of the superfamily of ras-related proteins (11). The tryptic radioactive peptide had the sequence lys-lys-ser-ser that localizes the phosphorylation site to the carboxyterminal end at serine 179 and/or serine 180, which

TABLE 2. *Carboxy-terminal amino acids of human ras and rap1 proteins*

H-ras	Met	Ser	Cys	Lys	Cys	Val	Leu	Ser
N-ras	Met	Gly	Leu	Pro	Cys	Val	Val	Met
rap1A	Lys	Lys	Lys	Ser	Cys	Leu	Leu	Leu
rap IB	Lys	Lys	Ser*	Ser*	Cys	Gln	Leu	Leu

Note: Cys in ras- and probably in rap- proteins, too, becomes carboxy-terminal, carboxymethylated, and farnesylated through posttranslational modifications. * Indicates the possible phosphorylation sites for protein kinase A.

are in direct vicinity to cysteine 181 (Table 2). It is known that P21 ras proteins undergo extensive posttranslational modifications at their carboxy-terminal end: the carboxyterminal three amino acids are cleaved proteolytically, and cysteine, which is then carboxy-terminal, becomes carboxymethylated and farnesylated (12). These modifications are essential for the membrane insertion and function of ras P21 proteins (13). It is likely that rap proteins undergo a similar series of posttranslational modifications. This is supported by the observed hydrophobicity of the isolated carboxy-terminal peptides of rap1B. Also, no amino acid sequence could be obtained beyond serine 180 of rap1B indicating that the terminal cysteine might be blocked by posttranslational modification.

At present, the function of rap1B is not known. Rap1B is 95% homologous with rap1A (identical to Krev-1) that has been shown to reverse the transformed phenotype of ras-transformed cells (14). The antioncogenic potential of rap1B awaits further experimentation. Time-course studies show that phosphorylation of rap1B is not related to inhibition of phospholipase C and platelet activation (W. Siess, unpublished observations).

CONCLUSION

Cyclic AMP inhibits platelet activation in multiple steps: it inhibits receptor-mediated phosphoinositide hydrolysis by phospholipase C, Ca^{2+} mobilization, PKC activation, and fibrinogen receptor exposure, and it also inhibits secretion and aggregation at steps distal to Ca^{2+} mobilization and activation of PKC and Ca^{2+}-dependent kinases. The cyclic AMP–dependent phosphorylation of target proteins or enzymes involved in these steps is getting characterized. At present, the following proteins have been identified as substrates for protein kinase A in intact platelets: rap1B (22 kDa), the β-chain of glycoprotein Ib (24 kDa) (15), and actin-binding protein (250 kDa). Glycoprotein Ib binds thrombin and von Willebrand factor and interacts through actin-binding protein with the platelet cytoskeleton (2). The further structural and functional study of proteins phosphorylated by protein kinase A will provide important clues for the understanding of the molecular mechanisms of platelet activation.

ACKNOWLEDGMENTS

This work was supported by the Deutsche Forschungsgemeinschaft with a Heisenberg fellowship (274/3-2).

REFERENCES

1. Moncada S, Gryglewski R, Bunting S, Vane JR. An enzyme isolated from arteries transforms prostaglandin endoperoxides to an unstable substance that inhibits platelet aggregation. *Nature* 1976;263:663–665.
2. Siess W. Molecular mechanisms of platelet activation. *Physiol Rev* 1989;69:58–178.
3. Siess W, Lapetina EG. Prostacyclin inhibits platelet aggregation induced by phorbol ester or Ca^{2+}-ionophore at steps distal to activation of protein kinase C and Ca^{2+}-dependent protein kinases. *Biochem J* 1989;258:57–65.
4. Bushfield M, McNicol A, MacIntyre DE. Inhibition of platelet-activating-factor-induced human platelet activation by prostaglandin D_2. *Biochem J* 1985;232:267–271.
5. Siess W, Lapetina EG. Phorbol esters sensitize platelets to activation by physiological agonists. *Blood* 1987;70:1373–1381.
6. Siess W, Lapetina EG. Ca^{2+}-mobilization primes protein kinase C in human platelets. *Biochem J* 1988;255:309–18.
7. Fischer TH, White GC. cAMP-dependent protein kinase substrates in platelets. *Biochem Biophys Res Commun* 1989;159:644–650.
8. Käser-Glanzmann R, Gerber E, Lüscher EF. Regulation of the intracellular calcium levels in human blood platelets: cyclic adenosine 3',5'-monophosphate dependent phosphorylation of a 22,000 dalton component in isolated Ca^{2+}-accumulating vesicles. *Biochim Biophys Acta* 1979;558:344–347.
9. Winegar DA, Siess W, Reep B, Ohmstede C, Lapetina EG. *Rap*1B is phosphorylated by cAMP-dependent protein kinase in intact human platelets. (Submitted for publication).
10. Lapetina EG, Lacal JC, Reep BR, Molina y Vedia L. A *ras*-related protein is phosphorylated and translocated by agonists that increase cAMP levels in human platelets. *Proc Natl Acad Sci* 1989;86:3131–3134.
11. Pizon V, Chardin P, Lerosey I, Olofsson B, Tavitian A. Human cDNAs *rap*1 and *rap*2 homologous to the Drosophila gene Dras3 encode proteins closely related to ras in the 'effector' region. *Oncogene* 1988;3:201–204.
12. Lowy DR, Willumsen BM. New clue to the *ras*-lipid glue. *Nature* 1989;341:384–385.
13. Barbacid M. *Ras* genes. *Annu Rev Biochem* 1987;56:779–827.
14. Kitayama H, Sugimoto Y, Matsuzaki T, Ikawa Y, Noda M. A *ras*-related gene with transformation suppressor activity. *Cell* 1989;56:77–84.
15. Wardell MH, Reynolds CC, Berndt MC, Wallace RW, Fox JEB. Platelet glycoprotein Ibβ is phosphorylated on serine 166 by cyclic AMP-dependent protein kinase. *J Biol Chem* 1989;264:15656–15661.

Atherosclerosis Reviews, Volume 21,
edited by A. Leaf and P. C. Weber.
Raven Press, Ltd., New York © 1990.

Platelet–Vessel Wall Interactions

Platelet Adhesion and Aggregation

Jacek Hawiger

Division of Experimental Medicine, New England Deaconess Hospital,
Boston, Massachusetts 02215

The interaction of platelets with the vessel wall provides the first line of defense against hemorrhage. Physiologic hemostasis is essential for the arrest of bleeding due to accidental or surgical cuts. Pathological thrombi are formed in response to endothelial injury and detachment resulting in exposure of the thrombogenic subendothelial extracellular matrix. Thrombotic occlusion of coronary and cerebral arteries is responsible for acute myocardial infarction and stroke, which contributed to over 566,000 and 147,000 deaths, respectively, in the U.S. in 1986 (1). So far, the pathologic formation of thrombi composed of platelets and fibrin seems to be similar to the formation of hemostatic platelet-fibrin thrombi (2,3).

The interaction of platelets with an atherosclerotic plaque, most likely upon its rupture, is the most frequent underlying cause of the thrombotic occlusion of coronary and cerebral arteries. The exact mechanism of interaction of platelets with an atherosclerotic plaque and the role of cellular and intercellular adhesion molecules still are understood poorly. The substantial rate (12–48%) of reocclusion of coronary arteries, following thrombolytic therapy and translumenal coronary angioplasty (4), indicates that formation of platelet and fibrin thrombi takes place even in those patients who continue to receive heparin and/or platelet inhibitors, such as aspirin.

This process, illustrated in Fig. 1, can be divided into the following stages. First, a zone of vascular injury is recognized by platelets that come into contact, change shape from smooth discs into spiny spheres, and spread. Second, more platelets are attracted to the area, their activation is manifest by secretion and degranulation that transforms them into "empty balloons," and results in adherence to each other to form a platelet thrombus (or a primary hemostatic plug when a vessel wall is cut). Third, thrombin is generated and can be detected within 45 sec (5). Thrombin activates platelets and transforms fibrinogen into fibrin polymer enmeshing platelets like a cocoon. Thus, a platelet–fibrin thrombus or a secondary hemostatic plug is formed that is more resistant to the shear

BEFORE ENDOTHELIAL INJURY   ENDOTHELIAL INJURY   PLATELET THROMBUS   PLATELET-FIBRIN THROMBUS

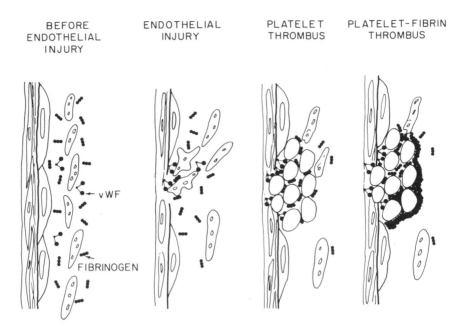

FIG. 1. Formation of platelet-fibrin thrombi. von Willebrand Factor serves as an anchor mediating adhesion of platelets to the zone of vascular injury. Fibrinogen plays a dual role as an adhesive molecule bridging the receptor (GPIIb–IIIa) on activated platelets and a second role as a substrate for thrombin. The resulting fibrin meshwork constitutes an integral structure of the platelet–fibrin thrombus.

stress of the blood flow. The arrest of bleeding (physiological hemostasis) and the formation of vaso-occlusive thrombi (pathological thrombosis) have a common denominator, namely, platelets adhere and aggregate "on demand" to form a thrombus (6).

Experimentally, the endothelium can be stripped from the inner aspect of the blood vessel in the system developed by Baumgartner and colleagues (7). It consists of de-endothelialized, everted blood vessels, such as rabbit aorta or human renal artery, placed in an annular perfusion chamber through which freshly drawn blood is pumped under controlled flow conditions. The three steps of adhesive interactions of platelets with the subendothelium, i.e., contact, spreading, and platelet thrombus formation can be measured. The initial contact of a platelet through a few portions of the ruffled membrane is mediated by the interaction of the platelet glycoprotein Ib (GPIb complex) depicted in Fig. 2, with an adhesive molecule in the subendothelial extracellular matrix, von Willebrand Factor (vWF), under high-flow/high-shear conditions. Under low-flow/low-shear conditions, the interaction of other platelet receptors [possibly GPIa–IIa complex and GPIc–IIa complex corresponding to very late antigen-2 (VLA-2) and VLA-5] with the components of the extracellular matrix (collagen and fibronectin, respectively) is involved (8). A deficiency of the platelet mem-

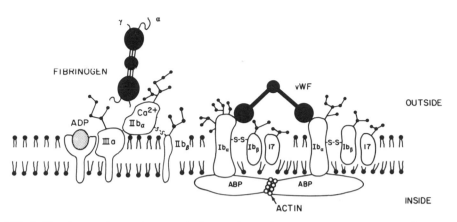

FIG. 2. Platelet membrane glycoprotein Ib complex and glycoprotein IIb–IIIa complex involved in their interaction with vWF and with fibrinogen.

brane glycoprotein Ib complex in giant platelet syndrome (Bernard–Soulier syndrome) leads to their inability to contact properly the zone of vascular injury (9).

The spreading of platelets involves the cytoskeletal apparatus, which becomes activated while platelets change shape from discoid forms into spiny spheres. Blocking the vWF in the subendothelial layer by antibody prevents contact and spreading of platelets *in vitro* (10). Spreading of platelets also is mediated by platelet glycoprotein IIb–IIIa (GPIIb–IIIa) interacting with adhesive molecules in the extracellular matrix, vWF, vitronectin, and possibly fibronectin (for review, see ref. 5). Platelet spreading is impaired in congenital deficiency of GPIIb–IIIa complex (Glanzmann's thrombasthenia) or when monoclonal antibodies are used against the GPIIb IIIa complex or synthetic peptides known to block binding of adhesive molecules to GPIIb–IIIa (11,12).

Thrombus formation depends on the bridging of platelets by fibrinogen derived from plasma or from platelet α granules and the interacting with activated platelets via the GPIIb–IIIa complex. Thus, under normal conditions a platelet thrombus is spanned by interplatelet bridges formed by fibrinogen. In the absence of plasma and platelet fibrinogen, other adhesive proteins, most likely vWF, are capable of mediating platelet thrombus formation (12–14). The central event in the formation of platelet thrombi is the transition of platelet receptors from the "nonbinding" to the "binding" mode, or from the nonactivated to the activated state. This transition results in the rearrangement of platelet GPIIb–IIIa in such a way that fibrinogen is recognized as depicted in Fig. 3. Adhesion of platelets to vascular shunts is mediated, at least in part, by fibrinogen deposited thereon (15). Polymerized fibrinogen on the surface or in solution appears to have more adhesive properties than native fibrinogen and may require only subthreshold activation of platelets (16).

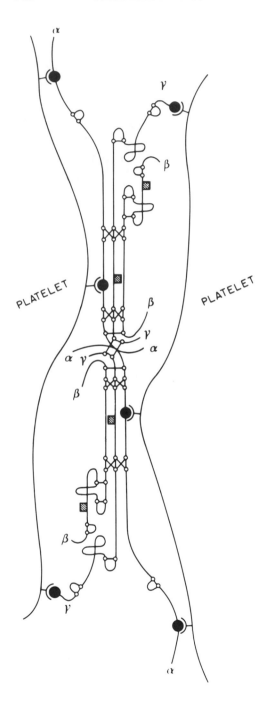

FIG. 3. Model depicting points of contact (filled circles) (receptor-recognition domains) on human fibrinogen involved in its interaction with platelets. Platelet receptors for fibrinogen comprise glycoprotein IIb–IIIa complexes switched to the binding mode during platelet activation. From ref. 103.

ADHESIVE MOLECULES MEDIATING THE INTERACTION OF PLATELETS WITH THE VESSEL WALL

The currently known adhesive molecules that mediate the interaction of platelets with the vessel wall can be divided into three classes depending on their localization and function (Table 1). Hence, adhesive molecules expressed on the platelet membrane belong to a family of cell adhesion molecules (CAMs) called also integrins (5,17,18). They function as receptors for other adhesive molecules present in plasma and in the extracellular matrix. The platelet membrane GPIIb–IIIa complex is a prime example of the "integrin" family of cell adhesion molecules. Adhesive molecules present in plasma or secreted into the plasma from platelet α granules belong to a class of intercellular adhesion molecules (IAMs) and they function as ligands in the fluid phase. Fibrinogen is the prime example of an IAM. Adhesive molecules deposited in the extracellular matrix, dubbed as matrix adhesion molecules (MAMs), function as ligands in the solid phase. The prime examples are vWF, fibronectin, and collagen. Some of them utilize sequence Arg-Gly-Asp (RGD) as a primary site of recognition specificity toward integrins (18).

von Willebrand Factor

vWF (subunit 240,000 Mr) is a multimeric glycoprotein synthesized in endothelial cells and stored therein in the Weibel–Palade bodies (19). It is secreted into the plasma and/or deposited in the subendothelial extracellular matrix. The multimers detectable in plasma range in size from 1 to 12 million Da (20). Another site of synthesis of vWF are megakaryocytes from which vWF ends up being packaged into platelet granules and secreted therefrom. Available data indicate that vWF secreted from platelet α granules has a higher proportion of large multimers than does plasma vWF (21). Although the gene for vWF has been cloned and the primary sequence of vWF has been unraveled recently (22), the structural features of vWF multimers present in plasma and in the

TABLE 1. *Cellular, intercellular, and matrix adhesion molecules at the platelet-vessel wall interphase*

Cell adhesion molecules (CAMs)	Intercellular adhesion molecules (IAMs)	Matrix adhesion molecules (MAMs)
GP Ib complex	von Willebrand factor (vWF)	vWF
GP IIb–IIIa complex	Fibrinogen, vitronectin, fibronectin	Fibronectin, vitronectin
GP Ia–IIa complex (VLA-2)		Collagen
GP Ic–IIa complex (VLA-5)	Fibronectin	Fibronectin
GP Ic–IIa complex (VLA-6)		Laminin
GP IV	Thrombospondin	Thrombospondin
Function: Receptors for IAMs, MAMs	Function: Ligands in fluid phase	Function: Ligands in solid phase

subendothelium that determine their potential difference in reactivity toward platelet receptors, are still unclear (23). The amino-terminal segment of the vWF subunit between residues Val^{449}-Lys^{728} contains two receptor recognition domains for GPIb (Cys^{474}-Pro^{488} and Leu^{694}-Pro^{708}) separated by a 205 residue segment (24). Ristocetin, which is known to modify the net charge of the platelet membrane, appears to "unlock" the GPIb binding domain for vWF or the vWF site for GPIb. Such a preparatory step is not always necessary because modified vWF (asialo vWF) or vWF present in patients with type IIb von Wille-brand disease interacts with platelet GPIb in the absence of ristocetin (25–28). It is noteworthy that the fibrin monomer promotes the interaction of vWF with human platelet GPIb, thereby providing a functional link between thrombin-induced clotting of fibrinogen and the binding of vWF to GPIb (29). Moreover, stress-induced aggregation of human platelets is mediated by vWF multimers present in plasma (30).

Platelets from patients with Bernard–Soulier syndrome that are deficient in the GPIb complex (3) do not bind vWF in the presence of ristocetin (31). Experiments with monoclonal antibodies directed against binding epitopes on glycoprotein Ib extended and confirmed these observations on the role of glycoprotein Ib as the platelet receptor involved in the binding of vWF by way of the classic mechanism (32). The GPIb is composed of two subunits, α and β, linked by a disulfide bond (Fig. 3). The primary structure of $GPIb_\alpha$ was elucidated by amino acid and cDNA sequencing (33,34). The location of a domain complementary to the receptor recognition domains of vWF is attributed to the amino terminal region of glycocalicin, a heavily glycosylated extraplatelet segment of $GPIb_\alpha$ (35,36).

The alternative receptor pathway for binding of vWF to human platelets evolved from our observation that thrombin in very low concentrations (0.008 to 0.05 U/ml) promoted binding of vWF to platelet receptors (37). In contrast to ristocetin, exposure of vWF binding sites by thrombin required metabolically intact platelets, was blocked by divalent ion chelators (EDTA and EGTA), and was inhibited by PGI_2. Platelets from patients with Glanzmann's thrombasthenia, known to have a deficiency of glycoproteins IIb and IIIa, did not bind vWF after stimulation with thrombin (38). Monoclonal antibodies against the GPIIb–IIIa epitope blocked binding of vWF, thus reaffirming the role of GPIIb–IIIa in the receptor function of platelets (39). The synthetic dodecapeptide corresponding to the carboxy-terminal segment of the human fibrinogen γ chain (γ 400–411) inhibited binding of vWF only when the "alternative" ADP-dependent receptor mechanism was involved (40). Similar results were observed in our and other laboratories with the synthetic peptide RGDS, which was initially identified as an analog of the cell-adhesion site of fibronectin fragment IV, and of the sequence 1744 to 1747 present in human vWF (41,42). In the presence of 40 μM RGDS, complete inhibition of binding of vWF to ADP-treated human platelets and their aggregation was observed (13,43).

Moreover, two adhesive glycoproteins, vWF and fibrinogen, inhibited each other at the given concentrations in respect to their binding to the site(s) exposed on ADP-treated platelets (40). Binding of vWF to platelets stimulated with ADP was accompanied by their aggregation in the absence of other plasma proteins, in particular fibrinogen, when the vWF concentration reaches values exceeding 30 μg (13). Thus, vWF not only participates in the adhesion of platelets through the subendothelial extracellular matrix, necessary for anchoring of platelets, but it may contribute to the formation of interplatelet linkages necessary for thrombus formation.

Collagen

When adhesion of platelets to the subendothelium was studied in Baumgartner's model (under condition of low shear when the presence of vWF is not essential) collagen was involved most prominently in contact with platelets, after other components of the extracellular matrix were degraded with α-chymotrypsin (44). Initially, collagen type I, the α_1 chain, was used to isolate receptors from the platelet membrane by affinity chromatography (45). The reported Mr of the collagen α_1 (I) receptor was 65,000, a distinctly lower molecular weight than was either the platelet membrane glycoprotein GPIa–IIa complex or the GPIIb–IIIa complex subsequently shown to be involved in the interaction of platelets with collagen (46–51). The nine residue sequence Gly-Lys-Hyp-Gly-Glu-Hyp-Gly-Pro-Lys from the cyanogen bromide–derived fragment, CN4, encompassing residues 403 to 551 of the α (III) chain, was proposed as an "adhesive site" of collagen (52). Subsequently, the nanopeptide corresponding to this sequence was shown to inhibit secretion of ^{14}C-serotonin induced by type III collagen, but to a lesser degree than if induced by type I collagen (53). Polyvalent interactions of collagen may contribute to the formation of much tighter bonds than individual fragments and peptides (54).

Fibronectins

Fibronectins are dimeric or multimeric molecules composed of subunits with an apparent Mr of 220,000. They are involved in various adhesive interactions occurring during embryonic development of tissues and organs, attachment of cells to extracellular matrix, wound healing, and possibly phagocytosis (55). Fibronectin is packaged into α granules of platelets and is secreted and bound to their membrane following activation with thrombin (56). Although the GPIIb–IIIa complex on platelets initially was thought to be a receptor for fibronectin (57,58), a more specific platelet receptor for fibronectin later was identified as VLA-5 associated with platelet membrane glycoproteins Ic and IIa (47,59). This receptor does not require prior activation of platelets to mediate their adhesion to fibronectin-coated surfaces (59).

The role of plasma and cellular fibronectin in the adhesive interactions of platelets remains unclear. On the one hand, polyclonal antibodies against fibronectin reduced platelet adhesion to the subendothelium in human umbilical arteries (60), and monoclonal antibodies against a fibronectin epitope, not present on other plasma proteins, inhibited aggregation of platelets induced with thrombin or ionophore A23187 (61). On the other hand, fibronectin failed to mediate the aggregation of normal human platelets (62), and a normal level of fibronectin failed to correct abnormal platelet aggregation and adhesion in afibrinogenemia and von Willebrand disease, respectively.

Thrombospondin

Thrombospondin is secreted from α granules of platelets upon their activation with thrombin; the secreted form of thrombospondin has a molecular weight of $420,000 \pm 20,000$ and is composed of three disulfide-bonded subunits of molecular weight 142,000, forming a tripartite "bola" figure (63–66). After it is released from platelet α granules by thrombin, thrombospondin becomes bound to the platelet membrane (67), where it may interact with heparin (68), other platelets (69,70), fibrinogen (71), fibrin (72), or the subendothelial extracellular matrix components, fibronectin and collagen (73,74). Thrombospondin is recognized by platelet membrane glycoprotein IV (75). Thrombospondin participates in the control of vascular smooth muscle growth (76) and in tissue repair following "crush injury" to the skeletal muscle (77).

Laminin

Another component of the subendothelial extracellular matrix and of the basement membrane, laminin, is a large glycoprotein composed of three subunits, one large subunit with an Mr of 400,000 and two smaller subunits with Mrs of 200,000 and 180,000, respectively, forming a cross that participates in adhesive interactions of various cells including neurons (78). Laminin attached to plastic surfaces promotes binding of platelets without their activation, which is different from that observed when surfaces were coated with fibronectin or with collagen (79). The binding of platelets to laminin was inhibited by antilaminin antibodies but remained unaffected by a 50,000-fold excess of the peptide RGDS, representing the cell-adhesion site of fibronectin. Such a concentration of peptide blocked 50% of the binding of platelets to the fibronectin-coated surface. Platelet membrane heterodimer VLA-6 composed of glycoprotein Ic and IIa serves as a receptor for laminin in nonactivated platelets (80). Other cells bind laminin to an integrin receptor that is insensitive to inhibition by RGD peptides (81).

Vitronectin

Vitronectin ("serum spreading factor," S protein) is a protein isolated from serum and associated with platelets (82,83). The affinity of vitronectin toward glass offers a potentially significant mechanism for the adhesion of platelets to artificial surfaces (82). By analogy to fibronectin, the RGD sequence (residues 45–48) in vitronectin (84) may represent the platelet-receptor recognition domain. The presence of a sequence analogous with somatomedin B suggests that vitronectin may be a source of this mitogenic factor (85). The platelet receptor for vitronectin is activation-dependent and related to the GPIIb–IIIa complex (86). The vitronectin receptor in endothelial cells takes part in their attachment to the extracellular matrix (87,88).

Matrix-adhesion molecules, i.e., vWF, fibronectin, thrombospondin, collagen, laminin, and vitronectin, interact with heparin-like glycosaminoglycans. Heparin-like molecules are attached to the protein carrier forming a proteoglycan, which is intercalated into the membrane of endothelial cells through hydrophobic segments (89). With the core protein intercalated into the membrane of one cell, the proteoglycan can bind through its polysaccharide chains to the matrix-adhesion molecules or to the receptor present at the surface of neighboring cells and thus mediate cell-adhesive interactions.

PLATELET AGGREGATION MEDIATED BY FIBRINOGEN AS A PROTOTYPE OF THE FORMATION OF PLATELET THROMBI

Key evidence for the role of fibrinogen in platelet function *in vivo* and *in vitro* was provided by "an experiment of nature," congenital afibrinogenemia (90,91). In fact, not only the fibrinogen, which is present in plasma, but also that which is stored in platelet α granules, is essential for aggregation of platelets activated with agents such as thrombin (92,93). Aggregation of platelets induced by ADP is accompanied by their binding of fibrinogen (94). In fact, the main role of platelet agonists such as ADP, epinephrine, or thrombin is to induce the exposure of binding sites for fibrinogen on the platelet membrane (for review, see ref. 5). Because thrombin is detectable within 45 sec when blood vessels are wounded (84), its role in mobilization of fibrinogen receptors on human platelets is important in the platelet–fibrinogen interaction. Fibrinogen's interaction with thrombin-activated platelets fulfills the criteria for specific, saturable, and reversible binding mediated by receptors that bind approximately 44,000 molecules by fibrinogen per platelet with an apparent dissociation constant (K_d) of 2×10^{-7} M (95). Because the plasma concentration of fibrinogen is approximately 50 times higher, it is apparent that even when its plasma level decreases to 5% of the normal value, it is still sufficient to saturate the available binding sites on platelets.

Human fibrinogen, a clottable and adhesive protein is composed of three pairs of nonidentical chains (α, β, and γ) linked by a series of disulfide bonds and arranged in three main structural domains: one central E and two distal D (96). We showed that both the γ chain and the α chain bear sites interacting with receptors on ADP-activated platelets (97). The essential role of the γ chain in the interaction of human fibrinogen with receptors on activated platelets has been established (for review, see ref. 6). The 12-mer, carboxy-terminal segment of the γ chain, encompassing residues 400–411, was pinpointed by us as the platelet receptor recognition domain. This was done through the use of a "native" peptide isolated from CNBr-cleaved human fibrinogen γ chain (98) and truncated synthetic peptides (99). Interestingly, human fibrinogen that contains either the elongated variant B or the γ chain, resulting from alternative splicing, has an impaired ability to interact with platelet receptors (100–102). These studies led to the realization that the continuous sequence of twelve amino acid residues between positions 400 and 411 in the predominant A variant of the γ chain of human fibrinogen is required for its interaction with human platelet receptors.

Following our findings that isolated α chains from human fibrinogen were reactive with ADP-activated platelets (97), we provided direct structural data for the functional role of sequences RGDF (α 95 to 98) and RGDS (α 572 to 575) in the interaction of human fibrinogen α chain with receptors on activated platelets (103). Both domains contain the sequence RGD, identified previously as "the cell-recognition site" of fibronectin (42). It appears that the γ-chain domain confers ligand specificity on human fibrinogen (104) and combined with the two alpha-chain domains provides for the optimal platelet-aggregating function of fibrinogen.

It is apparent then that one molecule of fibrinogen bridging two platelets is trivalent in regard to each platelet, assuring a higher affinity due to the higher than one valency level (6). Thus, the presence of three domains on each half of the fibrinogen molecule interacting with platelet receptors provides optimal conditions for tighter binding of fibrinogen to platelets and for their subsequent aggregation (Fig. 3). All three domains are prone to enzymatic attack by plasmin, which can cleave the bond Lys^{406}-Gln^{407} in the γ chain and clip off sequences containing RGD in the α chain (105).

The Receptor Function of Platelet Glycoprotein IIb–IIIa Complex in Formation of Platelet Thrombi

The 40,000 copies of GPIIb–IIIa complex available on one platelet serve as the receptor for fibrinogen (Fig. 2). The binding of fibrinogen to GPIIb–IIIa is Ca^{2+}-dependent and fulfills 1:1 stoichiometry (106–109). The genes for GPIIb–IIIa have been cloned and the amino acid sequence of both glycoproteins has been deduced (110,111). Both glycoproteins share structural homology with other membrane glycoproteins in the integrin superfamily; in particular, GPIIIa is highly homologous with the β subunit of the endothelial vitronectin receptor

(112,113). The GPIIb–IIIa complex is missing in patients with Glanzmann's thrombasthenia and such platelets do not bind fibrinogen (114,115). Furthermore, the GPIIb–IIIa complex is involved in the high-affinity binding of calcium (116); the binding of fibronectin, vWF, and vitronectin to thrombin-treated platelets (38,86,117); and the binding of collagen (108). Monoclonal antibodies against the GPIIb–IIIa complex block the binding of fibrinogen, vWF, and fibronectin (57).

The key step in the binding of fibrinogen to platelet GPIIb–IIIa is the shift from the nonbinding to the binding mode. Since fibrinogen with its binding domains for the platelet receptor is available all the time, the receptors are regulated by gating mechanisms controlling the access of bulky adhesive macromolecules. We proposed that activation of platelets with ADP and thrombin opens "the gate" that, in resting platelets, prevents access of bulky adhesive macromolecules to the receptor (GPIIb–IIIa) (6). "The gate" can be a part of the GPIIb–IIIa complex. Support for "the gate" hypothesis comes from experiments with proteolytic enzymes (chymotrypsin and pronase), which cleave portions of GPIIIa, and possibly GPIIb, allowing fibrinogen to bind to platelets without a need for ADP-mediated activation (119,120). Related evidence evolves from the use of the Fab fragment derived from the activation-dependent monoclonal antibody against GPIIb–IIIa. The Fab fragment (Mr 50,000) gains access to GPIIb–IIIa on nonactivated platelets, whereas the parent IgG molecule (Mr 150,000) is restrained from binding unless platelets are activated with ADP (121). Platelet activation induces *cis*-translocation of GPIIb–IIIa complexes, which arrange into clusters (122,123). Whether this is concordant with the "rain forest" hypothesis of Loftus and Albrecht (124), in which the platelet surface becomes more accessible, remains to be established.

The positive regulation of GPIIb–IIIa function as a fibrinogen receptor can be accomplished also through an ADP-independent pathway. This pathway involves cyclooxygenase, which generates prostaglandin endoperoxides G_2 and H_2 and are known to induce binding of fibrinogen to platelets (125,126). Lack of involvement of ADP was based on the use of ADP-removing enzymes or the application of ATP as a competitive inhibitor of the ADP receptor. Likewise, R_p and S_p diastereoisomers of adenosine 5'-0-(1-thiodiphosphate) [(R)-ADP-α-S and (S)-ADP-α-S] did not block the effect of a stable endoperoxide analog, 11-α,9-α-epoxymethane prostaglandin H_2 (127). However, both diastereoisomers inhibited ADP-induced platelet aggregation. Thus, it is clear that regulation of GPIIb–IIIa, leading to its switch from "nonbinding" to "binding" mode, can also proceed via an ADP-independent pathway mediated by prostaglandin endoperoxides. However, blocking this pathway with aspirin does not "disarm" platelet GPIIb–IIIa. In fact, many studies on ADP-induced binding of [^{125}I]fibrinogen were performed routinely on "aspirinated" platelets (128). In such platelets, ADP-induced changes must involve the ADP receptor and aspirin-insensitive pathways such as the protein kinase C pathway. Aspirin-insensitive pathways of platelet stimulation may contribute to the outcome of a vaso-occlusive phenomenon, because aspirin is 48% to 50% effective in the primary prevention of stroke and heart attacks (130,131). One of the aspirin-insensitive pathways is mediated by protein kinase C, a key signal transducer in platelets. Protein kinase C mediates a change in GPIIb–IIIa from a "nonbinding to binding mode" (132). Other reports also indicated a role for phorbol ester-activated protein kinase C in binding of fibrinogen to the platelet GPIIb–IIIa complex (133,134).

We have shown that this process is either prevented or reversed by cyclic AMP-mediated reactions, in as much as an increase in cAMP levels induced by prostacyclin (PGI$_2$) or a nonprostanoid inhibitor such as forskolin correlates with inhibition of binding of fibrinogen and vWF to activated platelets, which is paralleled by inhibition of platelet aggregation (37,95,135). Dibutyryl cyclic AMP inhibits binding of fibrinogen and vWF to ADP-or thrombin-activated platelets (37,135). Infusion of PGI$_2$ in humans slows down formation of a hemostatic plug as measured by bleeding time (136,137). PGI$_2$ also reduces the adhesive interaction of platelets with artificial surfaces (138). Clearly, receptors for adhesive proteins associated with the GPIIb–IIIa complex are not mobilized when platelet cyclic AMP rises. Whether such an excess of cyclic AMP can be attained under physiologic conditions to assure a lack of reactivity (nonthrombogenicity) of the vascular endothelium toward platelets is not certain.

Fibrinogen-Independent Aggregation of Human Platelets

The evidence favoring an essential role for fibrinogen in platelet-aggregate formation has been derived from *in vitro* experiments showing the lack of aggregation of ADP-treated platelets in the absence of plasma fibrinogen and from the observation in patients with afibrinogenemia (for review, see ref. 6). In some patients with afibrinogenemia, however, the formation of a platelet thrombus appears to be normal, suggesting that other proteins substitute for the aggregating function of fibrinogen (139). We have shown that vWF binds to ADP-treated normal platelets and mediates their aggregation (140). Furthermore, vWF and fibrinogen compete for the common ADP-dependent receptor mechanism on human platelets (40). More recently, *in vitro* aggregation of platelet-rich plasma from afibrinogenemic patients has been reported to depend on binding of vWF to platelet membrane glycoproteins IIb and IIIa (14). Thus, vWF can compensate for a deficiency of fibrinogen in mediating formation of interplatelet linkages after stimulation with ADP or thrombin. This provides a rational explanation for the formation of platelet aggregates *ex vivo* and *in vitro* in patients with congenital and acquired afibrinogenemia or hypofibrinogenemia.

Elevated levels of shear stress in small arteries and arterioles that are narrowed by atherosclerosis or vascular spasm lead to pathological platelet thrombi formation. Unusually large vWF multimers derived from stressed endothelial cells are exceptionally effective in mediating shear-induced platelet aggregation. The cone-plate viscometer in which controlled fluid-shear stress up to 800 dyn/cm^2 can be generated, was used to demonstrate that formation of platelet aggregates can be induced when the largest multimeric forms of vWF are added (30). Such forms are released from cultured endothelial cells and possibly from the vascular endothelium subjected to hemodynamic stress in the microcirculation. Similar observations were made in plasma from patients with congenital afibrinogenemia, as well as in a system in which platelet receptors for vWF, namely, GPIb and GPIIb–IIIa complexes, were blocked with appropriate monoclonal antibodies. The implication of those observations is that shear stress-induced platelet-aggregate formation is mediated by high molecular weight multimers of vWF through a receptor mechanism that is distinct from previously recognized pathways involving GPIb and GPIIb–IIIa (141). Although ADP is required, aspirin did not inhibit shear stress-induced platelet aggregation, indicating the role of aspirin-insensitive pathways of platelet stimulation in the binding of large vWF forms to platelets stressed by shear forces (142).

NEW INHIBITORS OF PLATELET-ADHESIVE INTERACTIONS

The interaction of platelets with the vessel wall and with each other can be inhibited partially by a limited number of drugs, such as aspirin and other nonsteroidal, anti-inflammatory agents. These agents block the cyclooxygenase pathway of platelet stimulation, but they cannot inhibit thrombus (aggregate) formation completely when the potency of the agonist, e.g., thrombin or collagen, is sufficiently high (129). Synthetic peptide analogs of platelet-receptor-recognition domains of human fibrinogen constitute a new class of inhibitors of platelet aggregation acting at the final step of platelet stimulation through several pathways (99). Simply, their target is the "exposed" binding site on the platelet membrane GPIIb–IIIa complex for fibrinogen, vWF, and other adhesive proteins. Their antiplatelet action requires further testing *in vivo* and in clinical trials, but currently available data indicate that the concept of a therapeutic blockade of platelet receptors for adhesive proteins is gaining significance.

So far the peptide γ 400–411 reversibly inhibited the formation of a hemostatic plug in a rabbit mesenteric artery (104). In related *ex vivo* experiments, using whole human blood pumped through a Baumgartner chamber at controlled flow conditions, the synthetic peptide γ 400–411 and peptide RGDS inhibited platelet thrombus formation. A control peptide was inactive *in vitro* and *ex vivo* (12). Thus, identification of the carboxy-terminal segment of the γ chain of human fibrinogen as a domain responsible for its interaction with receptors on activated platelets resulted in the development of analogs of the native sequence encompassing residues γ 400–411, and in application of anti-peptide antibody against γ 385–411 (99). This antibody is also effective in blocking the interaction of human platelets with fibrinogen absorbed to a synthetic polymer surface, whereas several monoclonal antibodies toward other epitopes of human fibrinogen were not inhibitory (143).

In addition to the γ-chain domain interacting with the GPIIb–IIIa complex on activated platelets, the α chain bears two domains (α 95–98) and (alpha 572–575) shown to interact with platelets (103). Both domains contain the RGD sequence. Interestingly, synthetic peptides patterned on the α-chain domains block the interaction of γ chains, and peptides patterned on the γ-chain domain block the interaction of α chains with activated platelets (144). This suggests that the platelet receptor associated with the GPIIb–IIIa complex is isospecific in regard to both α- and γ-chain domains. Practically, the mixture of both types of peptide has an additive rather than a synergistic effect on the inhibition of [^{125}I]fibrinogen binding to activated platelets (144,145). Synthetic peptide analogs containing sequence RGD inhibited platelet aggregation and binding of fibrinogen, vWF, and fibronectin to activated platelets (43,58,146–148).

Comparison of the *in vitro* inhibitory potency of dodecapeptide γ 400–411 and tetrapeptide RGDS indicates that the latter is approximately three times more potent toward platelets than is the former. However, the RGD sequence is present in hundreds of proteins, some of them nonadhesive. The inhibitory effect of tetrapeptide RGDS on the adhesive receptors in endothelial cells may have detrimental consequences on the integrity of the vascular endothelium *in vivo. In vitro,* a peptide containing the RGDS sequence caused detachment of human endothelial cells from the extracellular matrix (87,88). On the other hand, the dodecapeptide γ 400–411 has a sequence "unique" for fibrinogen and not detected in other adhesive proteins. To increase the inhibitory potency of the γ-chain-specific peptide, "hybrid" peptides encompassing the known features of both peptides were designed. The resulting "hybrid" peptides are more potent than the peptide γ 400–411, although they retain their structural attributes (144).

Monoclonal antibodies against the platelet membrane GPIIb–IIIa complex (e.g., 7E3) block the binding of fibrinogen and other adhesive proteins to platelets *in vitro* (109). They interfere with platelet spreading and thrombus formation *ex vivo* and with platelet-mediated occlusion of coronary arteries in dogs and Dacron vascular grafts in baboons (150,151). However, the interaction of monoclonal antibodies with human endothelial cells *in vitro,* resulting in detachment and exposure of the thrombogenic extracellular matrix (152), raises concerns about their potential side effects on the integrity of the vascular endothelium *in vivo.* Recently, two natural peptides containing the RGD sequence were identified in snake venoms of the green tree viper (trigramin) and the viper *Echis carinatus* (echistatin). Both blocked platelet membrane glycoproteins IIb–IIIa *in vitro* (153,154) and the formation of platelet thrombi in rat mesenteric artery (155).

An alternative approach to GPIIb–IIIa receptor blockade will be inhibition of ligands such as vWF, because its concentration in plasma is very low (10–15 μg/ml) in contrast to fibrinogen (2 to 4 mg/ml). Monoclonal antibody against vWF blocks coronary thrombosis in pigs (156). Aurin tricarboxilic acid inhibits the interaction of large multimeric forms of vWF with platelet glycoprotein Ib by forming a complex with the ligand rather than with the receptor (157).

SYNOPSIS OF PLATELET ADHESIVE INTERACTIONS

Thrombosis superimposed on atherosclerosis constitutes the chief mechanism of cardiovascular diseases. Blood platelets and fibrinogen provide the bulk of the thrombi; their formation is triggered by vascular and extravascular signals. Platelets are activated through at least three stimulatory pathways; only one is sensitive to inhibition by aspirin (cyclooxygenase). Aspirin-insensitive pathways, mediated by protein kinase C and myosin light-chain kinase, lead to a change of platelet shape with an attendant striking increase in their surface (pseudopods) followed by exposure of receptors for fibrinogen and von Willebrand Factor (vWF) on GPIIb–IIIa. Another receptor for vWF (GPIb) is independent of platelet activation and functions primarily in vessels with a high shear rate.

The blockade of platelet receptors for adhesive molecules, present in subendothelium and in plasma, circumvents the problem of platelet activation. However, platelet receptors exposed on GPIIb–IIIa share common structural features with the endothelial receptor for vitronectin. Thus, blockade of platelet GPIIb–IIIa with synthetic peptides containing the RGD sequence, or with certain monoclonal antibodies, may cause inadvertent detachment or prevent attachment of endothelial cells in a zone of vascular injury. The peptide analogs of human fibrinogen γ-chain sequence 400–411 possess high selectivity for platelet GPIIb–IIIa because they do not cause detachment of endothelial cells. Thus, endothelial growth in the zone of vascular injury following thrombolysis and/or angioplasty will go unperturbed. The blockade of platelet-adhesion receptors with platelet-selective peptides reduces the formation of platelet thrombi, and consequently rethrombosis. Step-by-step analysis of platelet-adhesive interactions not only helps to understand molecular mechanisms of thrombosis and rethrombosis, but also helps to develop new classes of antithrombotic drugs.

ACKNOWLEDGMENTS

Studies conducted in the author's laboratory described in this chapter were supported by NIH Grants HL-30648 and HL-33014, from the National Heart, Lung and Blood Institute.

REFERENCES

1. U.S. Bureau of Health Statistics, 1987.
2. French JE, Macfarlane RG, Sanders AG. The structure of haemostatic plugs and experimental thrombi in small arteries. *Br J Exp Pathol* 1964;45:467.
3. Sixma JS, Wester J. The hemostatic plug. *Semin Hematol* 1977;14:265–299.
4. Serruys PW, Luijten HE, Beatt KJ, et al. Incidence of restenosis after successful coronary angioplasty: a time-related phenomenon. A quantitative angiographic study in 342 consecutive patients at 1, 2, 3, and 4 months. *Circulation* 1988;77:361–371.
5. Teitel JM, Bauer KA, Lau HJ, Rosenberg RD. Studies of the prothrombin activation pathway utilizing radioimmunoassays for the F_2/F_{1+2} fragment and thrombin-antithrombin complex. *Blood* 1982;59:1086–1097.
6. Hawiger J. Adhesive interactions of blood cells and the vessel wall. In: Colman RW, Hirsh J, Marder VJ, Salzman EW, eds. *Hemostasis and thrombosis. Basic principles and clinical practice.* 2nd. ed. Philadelphia: JB Lippincott, 1987:182–218.
7. Sakariassen KS, Muggli R, Baumgartner HR. Measurement of platelet interaction with components of the vessel wall in flowing blood. In: Hawiger J, ed. *Platelets: receptors, adhesion, secretion. Part A. Methods in enzymology.* San Diego: Academic Press, 1989;169:37–70.
8. Weiss HJ, Turitto VT, Baumgartner HR. Effect of shear rate on platelet interaction with subendothelium in citrated and native blood. I. Shear rate-dependent decrease of adhesion in von Willebrand's disease and the Bernard-Soulier syndrome. *J Lab Clin Med* 1978;92:750–763.
9. Baumgartner HR, Tschopp TB, Weiss HJ. Platelet interaction with collagen fibrils in flowing blood. II. Impaired adhesion-aggregation in bleeding disorders. A comparison with subendothelium. *Thromb Haemost* 1977;37:17–28.
10. Turitto VT, Weiss HJ, Zimmerman TS, Sussman II. Factor VIII/von Willebrand factor in subendothelium mediates platelet adhesion. *Blood* 1985;65:823–831.
11. Lawrence JB, Gralnick HR. Monoclonal antibodies to the glycoprotein IIb/IIIa epitopes involved in adhesive protein binding: Effects on platelet spreading and ultrastructure on human arterial subendothelium. *J Lab Clin Med* 1987;109:495–503.
12. Weiss HJ, Hawiger J, Ruggeri ZM, Turitto VT, Thiagarajan P, Hoffman T. Fibrinogen-independent platelet adhesion and thrombus formation on subendothelium mediated by glycoprotein IIb–IIIa complex at high shear rate. *J Clin Invest* 1989;83:288–297.
13. Timmons S, Hawiger J. von Willebrand Factor can substitute for plasma fibrinogen in ADP-induced platelet aggregation. *Trans Assoc Am Physicians* 1986;94:226–235.
14. DeMarco L, Girolami A, Zimmerman TS, Ruggeri ZM. von Willebrand Factor interaction with the glycoprotein IIb/IIIa complex. Its role in platelet function as demonstrated in patients with congenital afibrinogenemia. *J Clin Invest* 1986;77:1272–1277.
15. Cooper SL, Young BR, Lelah MD. The physics and chemistry of protein surface interactions. In: Salzman EW, ed. *Interaction of the blood with natural and artificial surfaces.* New York: Marcel Dekker, 1985:1–36.
16. McManama G, Lindon JN, Kloczewiak M, et al. Platelet aggregation by fibrinogen polymers crosslinked across the E domain. *Blood* 1986;68:363–371.
17. Hynes RO. Integrins. A family of cell surface receptors. *Cell* 1987;48:549–554.
18. Ruoslahti E, Pierschbacher MD. New perspectives in cell adhesion: RGD and intrgrins. *Science* 1987;238:491–497.
19. Wagner DD, Olmsted JB, Marder VJ. Immunolocalization of von Willebrand protein in Weibel-Palade bodies of human endothelial cells. *J Cell Biol* 1982;95:355–360.
20. Hoyer LW. The Factor VIII complex: structure and function. *Blood* 1981;58:1–13.
21. Lopez-Fernandez MF, Ginsberg MH, Ruggeri ZM, Batille FJ, Zimmerman TS. Multimeric structure of platelet factor VIII/von Willebrand Factor: the presence of larger multimers and their reassociation with thrombin-stimulated platelets. *Blood* 1982;60:1132–1138.
22. Sadler JE. The molecular biology of von Willebrand factor. *Thromb Haemost* 1987:61–79.
23. Chopek MW, Girma J-P, Fujikawa K, Davie EW, Titani K. Human von Willebrand Factor: a multivalent protein composed of identical subunits. *Biochemistry* 1986;3146–3155.
24. Mjohri H, Fujimura Y, Shima M, et al. Structure of the von Willebrand Factor domain interacting with glycoprotein Ib. *J Biol Chem* 1988;263:17901–17904.
25. DeMarco L, Shaprio SS. Properties of human asialo factor VIII. A ristocetin-independent platelet-aggregatory agent. *J Clin Invest* 1981;68:321–328.

26. Gralnick HR, Williams SB, Coller BS. Asialo von Willebrand Factor interactions with platelets. *J Clin Invest* 1985;75:19–25.
27. DeMarco L, Girolami A, Russell S, Ruggeri ZM. Interaction of asialo von Willebrand Factor with glycoprotein Ib induces fibrinogen binding to the glycoprotein IIb/IIIa complex and mediates platelet aggregation. *J Clin Invest* 1985;75:1198–1203.
28. DeMarco L, Mazzuccato M, Grazia DBM, et al. Type IIB von Willebrand Factor with normal sialic acid content induces platelet aggregation in the absence of ristocetin. Role of platelet activation, fibrinogen, and two distinct membrane receptors. *J Clin Invest* 1987;80:475–482.
29. Loscalzo J, Inbal A, Handin RI. von Willebrand protein facilitates platelet incorporation in polymerizing fibrin. *J Clin Invest* 1986;78:1112–1119.
30. Moake JL, Turner NA, Stathopoulos NA, Nolasco LH, Hellums JD. Involvement of large plasma von Willebrand Factor (vWF) multimers and unusually large vWF forms derived from endothelial cells in shear stress-induced platelet aggregation. *J Clin Invest* 1986;78:1456–1461.
31. Moake JL, Olson JD, Troll JH, Tang SS, Funicella T, Peterson DM. Binding of radioiodinated human von Willebrand Factor to Bernard-Soulier, thrombasthenic and von Willebrand's disease platelets. *Thromb Res* 1980;19:21–27.
32. Coller BS, Peerschke EI, Scudder LE, Sullivan CA. Studies with a murine monoclonal antibody that abolishes ristocetin-induced binding of von Willebrand Factor to platelets: additional evidence in support of GPIb as a platelet receptor for von Willebrand Factor. *Blood* 1983;61:99–110.
33. Titani K, Takio K, Handa M, Ruggeri ZM. Amino acid sequence of the von Willebrand factor-binding domain of platelet membrane glycoprotein Ib. *Proc Natl Acad Sci USA* 1987;84:5610–5614.
34. Lopez JA, Chung DW, Fujikawa K, Hagen FS, Papayannopoulou T, Roth GJ. Cloning of the alpha chain of human platelet glycoprotein Ib: A transmembrane protein with homology to leucine-rich alpha 2-glycoprotein. *Proc Natl Acad Sci USA* 1987;84:5615–5619.
35. Okamura T, Jamieson GA. Platelet glycocalicin: A single receptor for platelet aggregation induced by thrombin or ristocetin. *Thromb Res* 1976;8:701–706.
36. Vincente V, Kostel PJ, Ruggeri ZM. Isolation and functional characterization of the von Willebrand factor-binding domain located between residues His^1-Arg^{293} of the alpha-chain of glycoprotein Ib. *J Biol Chem* 1988;263:18473–18479.
37. Fujimoto T, Ohara S, Hawiger J. Thrombin-induced exposure and prostacyclin inhibition of the receptor for Factor VIII/von Willebrand Factor on human platelets. *J Clin Invest* 1982;69:1212–1222.
38. Ruggeri ZM, Bader R, DeMarco L. Glanzmann's thrombasthenia: deficient binding of von Willebrand Factor to thrombin-stimulated platelets. *Proc Natl Acad Sci USA* 1982;79:6038–6041.
39. Ruggeri ZM, DeMarco L, Gatti L, Bader R, Montgomery RR. Platelets have more than one binding site for von Willebrand factor. *J Clin Invest* 1983;72:1–12.
40. Timmons S, Kloczewiak M, Hawiger J. ADP-dependent common receptor mechanism for binding of von Willebrand factor and fibrinogen to human platelets. *Proc Natl Acad Sci USA* 1984;81:4935–4939.
41. Titani K, Kumer S, Takio K, et al. Amino acid sequence of human von Willebrand Factor. *Biochemistry* 1986;25:3171–3184.
42. Pierschbacher MD, Ruoslahti E. Cell attachment activity of fibronectin can be duplicated by small synthetic fragments of the molecule. *Nature* 1984;309:30–33.
43. Plow EF, Pierschbacher MD, Ruoslahti E, Marguerie G, Ginsberg MH. The effect of Arg-Gly-Asp-containing peptides on fibrinogen and von Willebrand Factor binding to platelets. *Proc Natl Acad Sci USA* 1985;82:8057–8061.
44. Baumgartner HR. Platelet interaction with collagen fibrils in flowing blood. I. Reaction of human platelets with alpha-chymotrypsin-digested subendothelium. *Thromb Haemost* 1977;37:1–16.
45. Fauvel F, Legrand YJ. Inhibition of type III collagen induced platelet aggregation by active alpha-1 (III) CB4 peptide fragments. *Thromb Res* 1979;16:269–273.
46. Pischel KD, Bluestein HG, Woods VL Jr. Platelet glycoproteins Ia, Ic, and IIa are physicochemically indistinguishable from the very late activation antigens adhesion-related proteins of lymphocytes and other cell types. *J Clin Invest* 1988;81:505–513.

47. Hemler ME, Crouse C, Takada Y, Sonnenberg A. Multiple very late antigen (VLA) hetero-dimers on platelets. *J Biol Chem* 1988;263:7660–7665.
48. Santoro SA. Identification of a 160,000 dalton platelet membrane protein that mediates the initial divalent cation-dependent adhesion of platelets to collagen. *Cell* 1986;46:913–920.
49. Takada Y, Wayner EA, Carte WG, Hemler ME. Extracellular matrix receptors, ECMRII and ECMRI, for collagen and fibronectin correspond to VLA-2 and VLA-3 in the VLA family of heterodimers. *J Cell Biochem* 1988;37:385–393.
50. Nieuwenhuis HK, Sakariassen KS, Houdijk WPM, Nievelstein PFEM, Sixma JJ. Deficiency of platelet membrane glycoprotein Ia associated with a decreased platelet adhesion to subendothelium: a defect in platelet spreading. *Blood* 1986;68:692–695.
51. Kotite NJ, Staros JV, Cunningham LW. Interaction of specific platelet membrane proteins with collagen: evidence from chemical cross-linking. *Biochemistry* 1984;23:3099–3104.
52. Fauvel F, Legrand YJ, Kuhn K, Bentz H, Fietzek PP, Caen JP. Platelet adhesion to type III collagen: involvement of nine amino acids from alpha-1 (III) CB4 peptide. *Thromb Res* 1979;16:269–273.
53. Legrand YJ, Karniguian A, Le Francier P, Fauvel F, Caen JP. Evidence that a collagen-derived nonapeptide is a specific inhibitor of platelet-collagen interaction. *Biochem Biophys Res Commun* 1980;96:1579–1585.
54. Santoro SA, Cunningham LW. Collagen-mediated platelet aggregation. *J Clin Invest* 1977;60:1054–1060.
55. Hynes RO, Yamada KM. Fibronectins. Multifunctional modular glycoproteins. *J Cell Biol* 1982;95:369–377.
56. Ginsberg MH, Painter RG, Forsyth J, Birdwell C, Plow EF. Thrombin increases expression of fibronectin antigen on the platelet surface. *Proc Natl Acad Sci USA* 1980;77:1049–1053.
57. Plow EF, McEver RP, Coller BS, Woods VL Jr, Marguerie GA, Ginsberg MH. Related binding mechanisms for fibrinogen, fibronectin, von Willebrand Factor, and thrombospondin on thrombin-stimulated human platelets. *Blood* 1985;66:724–727.
58. Gardner JM, Hynes RO. Interaction of fibronectin with its receptor on platelets. *Cell* 1985;42:439–448.
59. Piotrowicz RS, Orchekowski RP, Nugent DJ, Yameda KY, Kunicki TJ. Glycoprotein Ic-IIa functions as an activation-independent fibronectin receptor on human platelets. *J Cell Biol* 1988;106:1359–1364.
60. Houdijk WPM, Sixma JJ. Fibronectin in artery subendothelium is important for platelet adhesion. *Blood* 1985;65:598–604.
61. Dixit VM, Haverstick DM, O'Rourke K, et al. Inhibition of platelet aggregation by a monoclonal antibody against human fibronectin. *Proc Natl Acad Sci USA* 1985;82:3844–3848.
62. Zucker MB, Mosesson MW, Brockman MJ, Kaplan KL. Release of platelet fibronectin (cold-insoluble globulin) from alpha granules induced by thrombin or collagen, lack of requirement for plasma fibronectin in ADP-induced platelet aggregation. *Blood* 1979;54:8.
63. Baenziger NL, Brodie GN, Majerus PW. A thrombin-sensitive protein of human platelet membranes. *Proc Natl Acad Sci USA* 1971;68:240–247.
64. Lawler JW, Slayter HS, Coligan JE. Isolation and characterization of a high molecular weight glycoprotein from human blood platelets. *J Biol Chem* 1978;253:8609–8616.
65. Coligan JE, Slayter HS. Structure of thrombospondin. *J Biol Chem* 1984;259:3944–3948.
66. Lawler J, Hynes RO. The structure of human thrombospondin, an adhesive glycoprotein with multiple calcium-binding sites and homologies with several different proteins. *J Cell Biol* 1986;103:1635–1648.
67. Phillips DR, Jennings LK, Prasanna HR. Ca^{2+}-mediated association of glycoprotein G (thrombin-sensitive protein thrombospondin). *J Biol Chem* 1980;255:11629–11632.
68. Slayter H, Karp G, Miller BE, Rosenberg RD. Binding properties of human thrombospondin: Interaction with mucopolysaccharides. *Semin Thromb Haemost* 1987;13:369–377.
69. Gartner TK, Williams DC, Minion FC, Phillips DR. Thrombin-induced platelet aggregation is mediated by a platelet plasma membrane-bound lectin. *Science* 1978;200:1281–1283.
70. Jaffe EA, Leung LLK, Nachman RL, Levin RI, Mosher DF. Thrombospondin is the endogenous lectin of human platelets. *Nature* 1982;295:246–248.
71. Leung LLK, Nachman RL. Complex formation of platelet thrombospondin with fibrinogen. *J Clin Invest* 1982;70:542–549.

72. Bale MD, Westrick LG, Mosher DF. Incorporation of thrombospondin into fibrin clots. *J Biol Chem* 1985;260:7502–7508.
73. Lahav J, Schwartz MA, Hynes RO. Analysis of platelet adhesion with a radioactive chemical cross-linking reagent: interaction of thrombospondin with fibronectin and collagen. *Cell* 1982;31:253–262.
74. Galvin NJ, Vance PM, Dixit VM, Fink B, Frazier WA. Interaction of human thrombospondin with types I-V collagen: direct binding and electron microscopy. *J Cell Biol* 1987;104:1413–1422.
75. Asch AS, Barnwell J, Silverstein RL, Nachman RL. Isolation of the thrombospondin membrane receptor. *J Clin Invest* 1987;79:1054–1061.
76. Majack RA, Cook SC, Bornstein P. Control of smooth muscle cell growth by components of the extracellular matrix; autocrine role for thrombospondin. *Proc Natl Acad Sci USA* 1986;83:9050–9054.
77. Watkins SC, Lynch G, Slayter HS. Thrombospondin is expressed in traumatized skeletal muscle: indication for a role in the repair of tissue. (Submitted for publication).
78. Timpl R. Structural and biological activity of basement membrane proteins. *Eur J Biochem* 1989;180:487–502.
79. Ill CR, Engvall E, Ruoslahti E. Adhesion of platelets to laminin in the absence of activation. *J Cell Biol* 1984;99:2140–2145.
80. Sonnenberg A, Modderman PW, Hogervorst F. Laminin receptor on platelets is the integrin VLA-6. *Nature* 1988;336:487–489.
81. Gehlsen KP, Dickerson K, Argraves WS, Engvall E, Rouslahti E. Subunit structure of a laminin-binding integrin and localization of its binding site on laminin. *J Biol Chem* 1989;264:19034–19038.
82. Barnes DW, Silnutzer J, See C, Shaffer M. Characterization of human serum spreading factor with monoclonal antibody. *Proc Natl Acad Sci USA* 1983;80:1362–1366.
83. Hayman EG, Pierschbacher MD, Ohgren Y, Ruoslahti E. Serum spreading factor (vitronectin) is present at the cell surface and in tissues. *Proc Natl Acad Sci USA* 1983;80:4003–4007.
84. Ruoslahti E, Suzuki S, Hayman EG, Ill CR. Purification and characterization of vitronectin. In: LW Cunningham, ed. *Structural and contractile proteins. Part D, Extracellular matrix.* Methods in Enzymology. San Diego: Academic Press, 1987;144:430–437.
85. Suzuki S, Pierschbacher M, Ruoslahti E. Domain structure of vitronectin: Alignment of active sites. *J Cell Biol* 1984;99:164a.
86. Thiagarajan P, Kelly KL. Exposure of binding sites for vitronectin on platelets following stimulation. *J Biol Chem* 1988;263:3035–3038.
87. Hayman EG, Pierschbacher MD, Ruoslahti E. Detachment of cells from culture substrate by soluble fibronectin peptides. *J Cell Biol* 1985;100:1948–1954.
88. Chen CS, Thiagarajan P, Schwartz SM, Harlan JM, Heimark RL. The platelet glycoprotein IIb/IIIa like protein in human endothelial cells promotes adhesion but not initial attachment to extracellular matrix. *J Cell Biol* 1987;105:1885–1892.
89. Marcum JA, Rosenberg RD. Heparin-like molecules with anticoagulant activity are synthesized by cultured endothelial cells. *Biochem Biophys Res Commun* 1985;126:365–372.
90. Inceman S, Caen J, Bernard J. Aggregation, adhesion, and viscous metamorphosis of platelets in congenital fibrinogen deficiencies. *J Lab Clin Med* 1966;68:21–32.
91. Weiss HJ, Rogers J. Fibrinogen and platelets in the primary arrest of bleeding. *N Engl J Med* 1971;285:369–374.
92. Morse EE, Jackson DP, Conley CL. Role of platelet fibrinogen in the reactions of platelets to thrombin. *J Clin Invest* 1965;44:809–819.
93. Tollefsen DM, Majerus PW. Inhibition of human platelet aggregation by monovalent antifibrinogen antibody fragments. *J Clin Invest* 1975;55:1259–1268.
94. Mustard JF, Packham MA, Kinlough-Rathbone RL, Perry DW, Regoeczi E. Fibrinogen and ADP-induced platelet aggregation. *Blood* 1978;52:453–466.
95. Hawiger J, Parkinson S, Timmons S. Prostacyclin inhibits mobilization of fibrinogen-binding sites on human ADP- and thrombin-treated platelets. *Nature* 1980;283:195–197.
96. Doolittle RF. Fibrinogen and fibrin. *Annu Rev Biochem* 1984;53:195–229.
97. Hawiger J, Timmons S, Kloczewiak M, Strong DD, Doolittle RF. Gamma and alpha chains of human fibrinogen possess sites reactive with human platelet receptors. *Proc Natl Acad Sci USA* 1982;79:2068–2071.
98. Kloczewiak M, Timmons S, Hawiger J. Localization of a site interacting with human platelet

receptor on carboxy-terminal segment of human fibrinogen gamma chain. *Biochem Biophys Res Commun* 1982;107:181–187.

99. Kloczewiak M, Timmons S, Lukas T, Hawiger J. Platelet receptor recognition site on human fibrinogen. Synthesis and structure-function relationship of peptides corresponding to the carboxy-terminal segment of the gamma chain. *Biochemistry* 1984;23:1767–1774.

100. Crabtree GR. The molecular biology of fibrinogen. In: Stamatoyannopoulos G, Nienhuis AW, Leder P, Majerus P, eds. *The molecular basis of blood diseases.* Philadelphia: WB Saunders, 1987:631–661.

101. Harfenist EJ, Packham MA, Mustard JF. Effects of variant gamma chains and sialic acid content of fibrinogen upon its interactions with ADP-stimulated human and rabbit platelets. *Blood* 1984;64:1163–1168.

102. Peerschke EI, Francis CW, Marder VJ. Fibrinogen binding to human blood platelets: Effect of gamma chain carboxy terminal structure and length. *Blood* 1986;67:385–390.

103. Hawiger J, Kloczewiak M, Bednarek MA, Timmons S. Platelet receptor recognition domains on the alpha chain of the human fibrinogen: structure function analysis. *Biochemistry* 1989;28:2909–2914.

104. Kloczewiak M, Timmons S, Bednarek MA, Sakon M, Hawiger J. Platelet receptor recognition domain on the gamma chain of human fibrinogen and its synthetic peptide analogs. *Biochemistry* 1989;28:2915–2919.

105. Doolittle RF. Fibrinogen and fibrin. In: Bloom AL, Thomas DP, eds. *Haemostasis and Thrombosis.* 1st ed. New York: Churchill Livingston. 1981:163–191.

106. Bennett JS, Vilaire G. Exposure of platelet fibrinogen receptors by ADP and epinephrine. *J Clin Invest* 1979;64:1393–1401.

107. Peerschke EI, Zucker MB, Grant RA, Egan JJ, Johnson MM. Correlation between fibrinogen binding to human platelets and platelet aggregability. *Blood* 1980;55:841–847.

108. Kornecki E, Niewiarowski S, Morinelli TA, Kloczewiak M. Effects of chymotrypsin and adenosine diphosphate on exposure of fibrinogen receptors on normal human and Glanzmann's thrombasthenic platelets. *J Biol Chem* 1981;256:5696–5701.

109. Coller BS, Peerschke EI, Scuder LE, Sullivan CA. A murine monoclonal antibody that completely blocks the binding of fibrinogen to platelets produces a thrombasthenic-like state in normal platelets and binds glycoproteins IIb and/or IIIa. *J Clin Invest* 1983;72:325–338.

110. Poncz M, Eisman R, Heidenreich R, et al. Structure of the platelet membrane glycoprotein IIb. *J Biol Chem* 1987;262:8476–8482.

111. Fitzgerald LA, Steiner B, Rall SC Jr, Lo S-S, Phillips DR. Protein sequence of endothelial glycoprotein IIIa derived from a cDNA clone. *J Biol Chem* 1987;262:3936–3939.

112. Fitzgerald LA, Poncz M, Steiner B, Rall SC Jr, Bennett JS, Phillips DR. Comparison of cDNA-derived protein sequences of the human fibronectin and vitronectin receptor alpha-subunits and platelet glycoprotein IIb. *Biochemistry* 1987;26:8158–8165.

113. Phillips DR, Charo IF, Parise LV, Fitzgerald LA. The platelet membrane glycoprotein IIb–IIIa complex. *Blood* 1988;71:831–843.

114. Nachman RL, Leung LLK. Complex formation of platelet membrane glycoproteins IIb and IIIa with fibrinogen. *J Clin Invest* 1982;69:263–269.

115. Bennett JS, Vilaire G, Cines DB. Identification of the fibrinogen receptor on human platelets by photoaffinity labeling. *J Biol Chem* 1982;257:8049–8054.

116. Brass LF, Shattil SJ. Identification and function of the high affinity binding sites for Ca^{++} on the surface of platelets. *J Clin Invest* 1984;73:626–632.

117. Ginsberg MH, Forsyth J, Lightsey A, Chediak J, Plow EF. Reduced surface expression and binding of fibronectin by thrombin-stimulated thrombasthenic platelets. *J Clin Invest* 1983;71:1–8.

118. Shadle PJ, Ginsberg MH, Plow EF, Barondes SH. Platelet-collagen adhesion: Inhibition by a monoclonal antibody that binds glycoprotein IIb. *J Cell Biol* 1984;99:2056–2060.

119. Greenberg JP, Orr JL, Packham MA, et al. The effect of pretreatment of human or rabbit platelets with chymotrypsin on their responses to human fibrinogen and aggregating agents. *Blood* 1979;54:753–765.

120. Niewiarowski S, Budzynski AZ, Morinelli TA, Brudzynski TM, Stewart GJ. Exposure of fibrinogen receptor on human platelets by proteolytic enzymes. *J Biol Chem* 1981;256:917–925.

121. Coller BS. Activation affects access to the platelet receptor for adhesive glycoproteins. *J Cell Biol* 1986;103:451–456.

122. Polley MJ, Leung LLK, Clark FY, Nachman RL. Thrombin-induced platelet membrane gly-

coprotein IIb and IIIa complex formation. An electron microscope study. *J Exp Med* 1981;154:1958.

123. Isenberg WM, McEver RP, Phillips DR, Shuman MA. The platelet fibrinogen receptor: an immunogold-surface replica study of agonist-induced ligand binding and receptor clustering. *J Cell Biol* 1987;104:1655–1663.

124. Loftus JC, Albrecht RM. Redistribution of the fibrinogen receptor of human platelets after surface activation. *J Cell Biol* 1984;99:822.

125. Bennett FS, Vilaire G, Burch JW. A role for prostaglandins and thromboxanes in the exposure of platelet fibrinogen receptors. *J Clin Invest* 1981;68:981–987.

126. Morinelli TA, Niewiarowski S, Kornecki E, Figures WR, Wachtfogel Y, Colman RW. Platelet aggregation and exposure of fibrinogen receptors by prostaglandin endoperoxide analogues. *Blood* 1983;61:41–49.

127. Cusack NJ, Hourani SMD. Effects of R_p and S_p diastereoisomers of adenosine 5'-O-(1-thiodiphosphate) on human platelets. *Br J Pharmacol* 1981;73:409–412.

128. Peerschke EI, Zucker MB, Grant RA, Egan JJ, Johnson MM. Correlation between fibrinogen binding to human platelets and platelet aggregability. *Blood* 1980;55:841–847.

129. Hawiger J, Steer ML, Salzman EW. Intracellular regulatory process in platelets. In: Colman RW, Hirsh J, Marder VJ, Salzman EW, eds. *Hemostasis and thrombosis. Basic principles and clinical practice.* 2nd edition. Philadelphia: JB Lippincott, 1987:710–725.

130. Gent M, Barnett HJM, Sackett DL, Taylor DW. A randomized trial of aspirin and sulfinpyrazone in patients with threatened stroke. Results and methodologic issues. *Circulation* 1980;62: V–97.

131. Preliminary report: Findings from the aspirin component of the ongoing physicians' health study. *N Engl J Med* 1988;318:262–264.

132. Timmons S, Tachiyama G, Hawiger J. The role of protein kinase C in the binding of fibrinogen and von Willebrand factor to the human platelet glycoprotein IIb–IIIa complex. (Submitted for publication.)

133. Shattil SF, Brass LF. Induction of the fibrinogen receptor on human platelets by intracellular mediators. *J Biol Chem* 1987;262:992–1000.

134. Niiya K, Hodson E, Bader R, et al. Increased surface expression of the membrane glycoprotein IIb/IIIa complex induced by platelet activation. Relationship to the binding of fibrinogen and platelet aggregation. *Blood* 1987;70:475–483.

135. Graber S, Hawiger J. Evidence that changes in platelet cyclic AMP levels regulate the fibrinogen receptor on human platelets. *J Biol Chem* 1982;257:14606–14609.

136. Gryglewski RJ, Szczeklik A, Nizankowski R. Anti-platelet action of intravenous infusion of prostacyclin in man. *Thromb Res* 1978;13:153–163.

137. FitzGerald GA, Miyamori LA, O'Grady J, Lewis PJ. A double blind placebo controlled evaluation of prostacyclin in man. *Life Sci* 1979;26:665–672.

138. Hawiger J, Graber S, Timmons S. Prostacyclin regulation of platelet receptors for adhesive macromolecules. In: Oates JA, Hawiger J, Ross R, eds. *Interaction of platelets with the vessel wall.* (Clinical physiology series.) American Physiological Society, 1985;89–102.

139. Turitto VT, Weiss HJ, Baumgartner HR. Platelet interaction with rabbit subendothelium in von Willebrand's disease: altered thrombus formation distinct from defective platelet adhesion. *J Clin Invest* 1984;74:1730–1741.

140. Fujimoto T, Hawiger J. Adenosine diphosphate induces binding of von Willebrand Factor to human platelets. *Nature* 1982;297:154–155.

141. Peterson DM, Stathopoulos NA, Giorgio TD, Hellums JD, Moake JL. Shear-induced platelet aggregation requires von Willebrand Factor and platelet membrane glycoproteins Ib and IIb-IIIa. *Blood* 1987;69:625–628.

142. Moake JL, Turner NA, Stathopoulos NA, Nolasco L, Hellums JD. Shear-induced platelet aggregation can be mediated by vWF released from platelets, as well as by exogenous large or unusually large vWF multimers, requires adenosine diphosphate, and is resistant to aspirin. *Blood* 1988;71:1366–1374.

143. Shiba E, Lindon J, Kushner L, et al. Changes in conformation of fibrinogen adsorbed on polymer surfaces detected by polyclonal and monoclonal antibodies. *Circulation* 1988;78:II–622.

144. Timmons S, Bednarek M, Kloczewiak M, Hawiger J. Antiplatelet "hybrid" peptides analogous to receptor recognition domains on gamma and alpha chains of human fibrinogen. *Biochemistry* 1989;28:2920–2923.

145. Bennett JS, Shattil SJ, Power JW, Gartner TK. Interaction of fibrinogen with its platelet receptor. *J Biol Chem* 1988;263:12948–12953.
146. Ginsberg M, Pierschbacher MD, Ruoslahti E, Marguerie G, Plow E. Inhibition of fibronectin binding to platelets by proteolytic fragments and synthetic peptides which support fibroblast adhesion. *J Biol Chem* 1985;260:3931–3936.
147. Ruggeri ZM, Houghten RA, Russell SR, Zimmerman TS. Inhibition of platelet function with synthetic peptides designed to be high-affinity antagonists of fibrinogen binding to platelets. *Proc Natl Acad Sci USA* 1986;83:5708–5712.
148. Plow EF, Pierschbacher MD, Ruoslahti E, Marguerie G, Ginsberg MH. Arginyl-Glycyl-Aspartic acid sequences and fibrinogen binding to platelets. *Blood* 1987;70:110–115.
149. Hayman EG, Pierschbacher MD, Ruoslahti E. Detachment of cells from culture substrate by soluble fibronectin peptides. *J Cell Biol* 1985;100:1948–1954.
150. Yasuda T, Gold HK, Fallon JT, et al. Monoclonal antibody against the platelet glycoprotein (GP)IIb/IIIa receptor prevents coronary artery reocclusion after reperfusion with recombinant tissue-type plasminogen activator in dogs. *J Clin Invest* 1988;81:1284–1291.
151. Hanson SR, Pareti FI, Ruggeri ZM, et al. Effects of monoclonal antibodies against the platelet glycoprotein IIb/IIIa complex on thrombosis and hemostasis in the baboon. *J Clin Invest* 1988;81:149–158.
152. Charo IF, Bekeart LS, Phillips DR. Platelet glycoprotein IIb–IIIa-like proteins mediate endothelial cell attachment to adhesive proteins and the extracellular matrix. *J Biol Chem* 1987;262:9935.
153. Huang T-F, Holt JC, Lukasiewicz H, Niewiarowski S. A low molecular weight peptide inhibiting fibrinogen interaction with platelet receptors expressed on glycoprotein IIb–IIIa complex. *J Biol Chem* 1987;262:16157–16163.
154. Gan Z-R, Gould RJ, Jacobs JW, Friedman PA, Polokoff MA. A potent platelet aggregation inhibitor from the venom of the viper, ECIS CARINATUS. *J Biol Chem* 1988;263:19827–19832.
155. Cook JC, Huang T-F, Rucinski B, Tuma RF, Williams JA, Niewiarowski S. Inhibition of platelet hemostatic plug formation by trigramin, a novel RGD containing peptide. *Circulation* 1988;78:II-313.
156. Bellinger DA, Nichols TC, Read MS, et al. Prevention of occlusive coronary artery thrombosis by a murine monoclonal antibody to porcine von Willebrand Factor. *Proc Natl Acad Sci USA* 1987;84:8100–8104.
157. Phillips MD, Moake JL, Nolasco L, Turner N. Aurin Tricarboxylic Acid: A novel inhibitor of the association of von Willebrand Factor and platelets. *Blood* 1988;72:1898–1903.

Atherosclerosis Reviews, Volume 21,
edited by A. Leaf and P. C. Weber.
Raven Press, Ltd., New York © 1990.

New Trends in Atherosclerosis Research

Agostino Faggiotto

Department of Pharmacology, Bayer-Italia, 20024 Garbagnate Milanese, Italy

In the early 1980s it was determined that one in every five adults over the age of 50 years would die of the complications of atherosclerosis (1,2). Although these projections did not take into account the negative trend of mortality for coronary heart disease (CHD) in the U.S. (3), the pathological manifestations of advanced atherosclerosis still take too many lives in our western population.

Furthermore, the average age of people belonging to the so-called industrialized world is steadily increasing, so that, in spite of a declining rate of CHD (which incidentally seems to be leveling off), we may expect to witness an increase in the incidence of symptomatic atherosclerosis in the years to come.

Many pharmaceutical companies, including ours, have become aware of these projections and are focusing their attention on atherosclerosis *per se* either by expanding their research capacities or by entering this area of research *de novo*. Their scientific approach to the treatment of this disease seems to have changed and some important therapeutic contributions in this field have been made already.

TREATING ATHEROSCLEROSIS

All of us have atherosclerosis in some form or another, although we may not be aware of its slow and silent progression. Certainly, if examined, we all could provide histological examples of focal, structural alterations in our larger arteries, which in time may evolve to become acutely or chronically symptomatic.

In January 1988 the Adult Treatment Panel Report appeared in the *Archives of Internal Medicine* (4). The report was concerned with the identification of high-risk individuals who could develop symptomatic atherosclerosis and benefit from intensive medical intervention.

The report deals with two basic questions: Who should be treated for high-blood cholesterol?; and How should they be treated (5)? This is similar to asking: *Who* should be treated for atherosclerosis? And *how?*

HOMEOSTATIC EQUILIBRIUM AND ENDOTHELIAL INJURY

Because arteries normally must withstand physiological stimuli, such as the pulsating pressure generated by the heart, daily changes in blood pressure, changes in blood composition, and changes in hormonal stimulation, within a biological range of stimulation the arterial response to such stimuli will cause no pathological outcome.

Possibly, the few adhering monocytes, the discrete numbers of foam cells, and the smooth-muscle-cell-rich intimal cell masses (ICM) found at branch sites of control animals and humans (6–8) testify that interactions between blood-borne cells and the cells of the arterial wall represent, within limits, a physiological response to biological stimuli.

Consequently, either the relative or absolute insufficiency of such homeostatic adaptive mechanisms or an exaggerated arterial reaction to stimulation will generate vascular disease.

Atherogenesis may represent the most common and relevant example of arterial response to sustained or episodic pathological vascular stimulation occurring over the years (9). Some of the best known proatherogenic factors are hypercholesterolemia, hypertension and flow disturbances, inflammation, oxidized or modified lipoproteins, smoking, diabetes, and stress.

In humans, many of these risk factors often coexist; the presence of multiple and interacting pathogenetic events seems to accelerate the progression of this disease. However, even the presence of a single risk factor could elicit a mixed array of biological phenomena interacting with more than one pathological event. For example, the presence of modified forms of low-density lipoprotein (LDL) has been documented in chronic diabetes (10,11); in addition, modified or oxidized intimal LDLs are capable of triggering a focal immune response in the intima, which includes the participation of T-lymphocytes, macrophages, and the activation of complement (12); among other effects, smoking, in itself, also may trigger an allergic reaction, which is likely to be based on the antigenic properties of tobacco glycoproteins (13,14).

TABLE 1. *The schematic progression of atherosclerotic lesions*

Normal structure
    Discrete focal numbers of adhering monocytes
    Some intimal foam cells
    Some intimal smooth muscle cells or intimal cell masses at bifurcations
Fatty streak
    Nonsymptomatic
    Predominant in young people
    Layers of foam cells
    Can regress (animal and human data)
    Can evolve to fibrous plaque
Fibrous plaque
    Many cellular and biochemical components are present and interacting
    Slowly reversible
    Can evolve to become complicated
Complicated lesion
    Often symptomatic
    Hardly reversible
    The "Killer"

In any case, the first cell that has to cope with any physiopathological stimulus is the endothelial cell. The results of sustained endothelial cell stimulation, or, in Virchow's words (15), "irritation," could lead to a number of effects, including: (a) increased endothelial cell turnover and (b) increased endothelial cell desquamation. Both of these are responsible for increased LDL uptake or modification, growth factor release in the intima, and smooth-muscle-cell chemotaxis and mitogenesis. (c) Adhesive endothelium is responsible for monolymphocyte adhesion, monolymphocyte infiltration into the intima, inflammatory phenomena, and macrophage activation, these, in turn, are responsible for foam cell formation, mitogen, cytokine release, and toxic macrophages.

The above-mentioned list is only a short and incomplete account of potential interacting atherogenic events that may occur focally in an artery and depicts only partially the complexity of atherogenesis at its onset and evolution. The main phases of atherosclerosis are outlined in Table 1.

NEW TRENDS

Clearly, atherosclerosis represents an extremely complex disease and different pathological processes such as inflammation, degeneration, and neoplasia are present and interact in its evolution; in addition, its onset and progression are very subtle, slow and silent, overlapping often with normal aging processes.

Today, in spite of a tremendous quantity of accumulated information, we can provide only partial explanations as to why atherosclerosis is so common in Western civilization, what is the reason for the presence of fatty streaks in young people, what is responsible for the conversion of fatty streaks to fibrous plaques, what is the role of inflammation in atherosclerosis, as reflected by the presence of T-8 lymphocytes in the intima, and by the monocyte–lymphocyte interaction within the arterial wall.

Eventually, when atherosclerosis becomes symptomatic, the treatment of choice often resorts to surgical procedures, as medical intervention has little or no short-term usefulness unless patients are subjected to a relatively long-term and aggressive therapy (16).

In the past, therapeutic research and development aimed at the complications of atherosclerosis; that is, why antithrombotic, antiplatelet, or anti-any risk factor therapics were and are being used or developed. Although in the end atherosclerosis *per se* is not the killer, but the complications of atherosclerosis plaques are responsible for the greatest part of the most dramatic medical emergencies, a number of pharmaceutical companies, including ours, have developed new R & D strategies aimed at inhibiting the onset and progression of nonsymptomatic atherosclerosis or at favoring the regression of its early lesions with more conventional forms of therapy.

Obviously, the sooner a therapeutical intervention, the better the chances of inducing effective regression and, perhaps also, the less complicated the biologi-

TABLE 2. *Three main population targets who could benefit from antiatherosclerosis education*

Group A	
Prevention of atherosclerosis development	New target
Group B	
Therapy of nonsymptomatic atherosclerosis	New target
Group C	
Therapy of symptomatic atherosclerosis	Old target

cal picture with which we are asked to interfere. At the same time, we should not interfere with those mechanisms that are necessary for the maintenance of our vascular homeostasis.

THEORETICAL STRATEGY FOR
A THERAPEUTICAL DEVELOPMENT

In theory, one could develop a strategy of drug development by examining the evolution of atherosclerosis, as schematically outlined in Table 1, and determining who could be the recipient of antiatherosclerosis therapy. Three main population targets could be proposed.

A first group (Group A) could be made of people who would benefit from all those approaches and procedures aimed at preventing the development of lesions; a second group (Group B) could include people with nonsymptomatic atherosclerosis, and, finally, in the third group (Group C) we could consider those people who already have clear signs and symptoms of atherosclerosis (Table 2). All three groups could benefit from enhanced antiatherosclerosis education, including changes in diet and lifestyle.

People belonging to Group A (that is, those who have no overt symptoms) could undergo screening procedures aimed at determining the relative risk for the development of premature atherosclerosis and, thus, potentially require the use of new antiatherosclerotic therapies.

Although the therapeutic approach for people belonging to Group C is aimed at the complications of atherosclerosis, by exploiting treatments such as thrombolitic, antiplatelet, spasmolitic or anti–any risk factor, the new pharmacological target is aimed mainly at people belonging to Group B, that is, at people who are known to be prone to atherosclerosis, but still have no symptoms of the disease.

Obviously, one needs to determine *who* is at greater risk and *what* are the atherogenic mechanisms that we are trying to inhibit.

EARLY ATHEROGENIC MECHANISMS

Observations made in several animals subjected to hypercholesterolemic diets have almost unequivocally given the same sequence of cellular and hu-

TABLE 3. *Schematic sequence of atherogenic events in the hypercholesterolemic animal (either fat-fed or LDL receptor negative)*

Hypercholesterolemia
Increased focal adhesion of monocytes to the endothelium
Infiltration of the intima by monocyte–macrophages
Lipid uptake by macrophages
Foam cell formation—endothelium still intact
Early smooth muscle presence in the intima
Exit of foam cells from the intima—EC retraction
Platelet adhesion to exposed subendothelial matrices
Development of proliferative lesions—fibrous plaque formation

moral events leading to experimental atherosclerosis. Recent accumulated knowledge would support the idea that animal models of experimental atherosclerosis and human atherosclerosis share many features, including the presence of modified forms of LDL in the intima of arteries (17).

The onset and evolution of atherosclerotic lesions, as observed in the hypercholesterolemic animal (either fat-fed or LDL-receptor negative), seem to follow this schematic series of events: First, with the progressive increase of cholesterolemia, one can observe the increased focal adhesion of leukocytes to an intact endothelium. Subsequently, leukocytes, believed to be mostly monocytes, infiltrate the intima and become tissue macrophages. There, intimal macrophages begin to take up lipid, eventually become engulfed with cholesteryl ester droplets and assume the appearance of foam cells. Fatty streaks are formed by several layers of juxtaposed multilayered lipidladen macrophages and represent the lesions of inception of atherosclerosis; the endothelium at this stage remains intact, although some macrophages were seen between endothelial cell junctions, as if in the process of leaving the arterial wall. It should be stressed that if cholesterolemia is brought back to normal levels, then the quantity and severity of these early lesions can be reduced drastically within a relatively short period of time. On the other hand, if hypercholesterolemia is maintained, some smooth muscle cells begin to appear in the intima and the endothelium begins to retract over the fatty streaks releasing foam cells in circulation and exposing intimal matrices to blood. Platelets adhere at these denuded sites and presumably release their granule content, as they normally would do in wound-healing processes. Frank proliferative lesions appear at this later stage and assume the appearance of fibrous plaques, regardless if the animal was fat-fed or was LDL-receptor negative (18–21) (Table 3).

PHARMACOLOGICAL TARGETS

Based on the considerations expressed above, let us now consider a number of salient atherogenic mechanisms best suited for pharmacological intervention and potentially bound to give the best positive outcome when influenced.

Screening programs would have to be carried out first in *in vitro* assays and cell culture systems, and then confirmed *in vivo* in the animal. Also, potential targets of therapeutical research could be aimed at testing specific experimental protocols mimicking aspects of atherosclerosis, including:

1. Antiadhesive substances for endothelium and leukocytes (?);
2. Substances that would prevent the lipid intake by macrophages, thus inhibiting foam cell formation (?). (Although it must be said that both targets represent a bit of a gamble, it still has to be determined when and how the monocyte–macrophage behaves as a "good" guy or a "bad" guy.);
3. Substances that would prevent lipoprotein modification (spontaneous or cell-mediated) and, thus, fatty streak formation;
4. Substances that would stimulate the reverse cholesterol transport (RCT) from the arterial wall to blood;
5. Substances that would increase the acceptor capacity for cholesterol esters, such as an increase in the plasma concentration of high-density lipoprotein (HDL), the natural acceptor for cholesterol esters;
6. New types of anti-inflammatory drugs against atherosclerosis, such as anti-T-8 activation; antimacrophages activation; and antilymphomonokine release; and
7. Antichemotactic, antimitogenic substances (perhaps heparin-like substances) for smooth muscle cells.

THERAPEUTIC TARGETS

Clearly, the new target today is to inhibit fatty streak formation, stimulate fatty streak regression, and inhibit the conversion of fatty streaks to fibrous plaques. However, there exist practical difficulties in the ways one would have to plan a clinical trial in a nonsymptomatic, relatively healthy population.

The population with short-term risk (Group C) is more attractive from the standpoint of a clinical trial, as it would be conceptually easier to prove the efficacy of a new drug within a short period of time. A group of such people could be represented by patients who have undergone endoarteriectomy or thromboangioplasty (PTCA).

However, the type, stage, and mechanisms of atherosclerosis between the nonsymptomatic target group and the group of people subjected to PTCA are quite different, and in theory a new drug could be ineffective in one group and effective in the other.

Pathogenetic differences of atherosclerosis between the two populations are represented by (a) a different type of arterial stimulation and response of the artery to stimuli; (b) the type of arterial cells involved in the response to stimulation are different and differently stimulated; and (c) the timing of lesion development is quite different.

Thus, how could we prove the efficacy of new experimental treatments tested in patients with advanced athero*sclerosis* + PTCA and be confident that they will work in patients with athero*genesis* in the making? The natural evolution of atherosclerosis is indicated below:

$$\begin{array}{cc} \text{R \& D target} & \text{Trial target} \\ \text{N} \rightarrow \quad \text{FS} \rightarrow \text{FP} \quad \rightarrow \text{CL} \rightarrow \text{CL} + \text{PTCA} \end{array}$$

It may be possible (according to recent data) to exploit biochemical markers for the presence of progressing atherosclerosis and look for young subjects with high levels of these markers. This approach would represent one way of selecting a small population of nonsymptomatic people at risk and study them in a follow-up program. Furthermore, it may be possible to use improved noninvasive techniques for the monitoring of those early silent atherosclerotic lesions in combination with or without a new drug.

Atherosclerosis is quite a complex disease and this simple outline only represents an input for further discussions. The development of a new drug requires many years of work and investment in pharmacological screening and testing with no clear guarantees on returns. This awareness underscores the importance of evaluating what the key atherogenic mechanisms are, how to reproduce them in the laboratory, how to interfere with them pharmacologically, how to determine who has the knowledge and the structures to carry out specific preclinical and clinical experiments, and how to favor the exchange of information between knowledge-based institutions and, from these interactions, finally to bring together a general plan of research and development for a new effective drug therapy specifically aimed at inhibiting the onset and progression of atherosclerosis.

REFERENCES

1. Report on the National Cholesterol Education Program expert panel on detection, evaluation, and treatment of high blood cholesterol in adults. *Arch Intern Med* 1988;251:365–374.
2. Stallones RA. The rise and fall of ischemic heart disease. *Sci Am* 1980;243:53–59.
3. Ahrens EH Jr, Connor WE, Bierman EL, et al. Report of the task force on the evidence relating six dietary factors to the nation's health. *Am J Clin Nutr* 1979;32(suppl 12):2621.
4. Goodman DS. Cholesterol revisited—Molecule, medicine, and media. [George Lyman Duff Memorial Lecture.] *Arteriosclerosis* 1989;9:430–438.
5. Report of the Working Group on Arteriosclerosis of the National Heart and Lung and Blood Institute, Washington, D.C.: U.S. vol. 2. Government Printing Office 1982:DHEW publication no. (NIH)82–2035).
6. Duff GL, McMillan GC, Ritchie AC. The morphology of early atherosclerotic lesions of the aorta demonstrated by the surface technique in rabbits fed cholesterol. Together with a description of the anatomy of the intima of the rabbit's aorta and the "spontaneous" lesions which occur in it. *Am J Pathol* 1957;33:845–861.
7. Geer JC, McGill HC, Strong JP. The fine structure of human atherosclerotic lesions. *Am J Pathol* 1961;38:263–287.
8. Oeser J, Fehr R, Brinkmann B. Aortic and coronary atherosclerosis in a Hamburg autoptic series. *Virchows Arch* [A] 1979;384:131–145.

9. Faggiotto A. Cellular dynamics in atherosclerosis. In: *Health Effects of Polyunsaturated Fatty Acids in Seafoods.* Simopolous AP, Kifer RR, Martin RE, eds. London: Academic Press, Inc. 1986:87–110.
10. Cerami C, Vlassara H, Brownlee M. Protein glycosilation and the pathogenesis of atherosclerosis. *Metabolism* 1985;34(suppl 1):37–44.
11. Lopes-Virella MF, Klein RL, Lyons TJ, Stevenson HC, Witztum JL. Glycosilation of Low Density Lipoprotein enhances cholesterol ester synthesis in Human-derived Macrophages. *Diabetes* 1988;37:550–57.
12. Hansson GK, Jonasson L, Seifert PS, Stemme S. Immune Mechanisms in Atherosclerosis. *Arteriosclerosis* 1989;9:567–578.
13. McGill HC Jr. Potential mechanisms for the augmentation of atherosclerosis and atherosclerotic disease by cigarette smoking. *Prev Med* 1979;8:390–403.
14. Turner DM. Carbon Monoxide, Tobacco Smoking, and the pathogenesis of Atherosclerosis. *Prev Med* 1979;8:303–309.
15. Brown GB, Lin JT, Schaefer SM, Kaplan CA, Dodge HT. Niacin or lovastatin, combined with colestipol, regress coronary atherosclerosis and prevent clinical events in men with elevated apolipoprotein B. *Circulation* 1989;80:II-266.
16. Virchow R. Der ateromatose Prozess der Arterien. *Wien Med Wochenschr* 1856;6:825–841.
17. Yla-Herttuala S, Palinski W, Rosenfeld ME, et al. Evidence for the presence of oxidately modified low density lipoprotein in atherosclerotic lesions of rabbit and man. *J Clin Invest* 1989;84: 1086–1095.
18. Faggiotto A, Ross R, Harker L. Studies of hypercholesterolemia in the non-human primate. I. Changes that lead to fatty streak formation. *Arteriosclerosis* 1984;4:323–340.
19. Faggiotto A, Ross R. Studies of hypercholesterolemia in the non-human primate. II. Fatty streak conversion to fibrous plaque. *Arteriosclerosis* 1984;4:341–356.
20. Rosenfeld ME, Tsukada T, Gown AM, Ross R. Fatty streak initiation in Watanabe heritable hyperlipemic and comparably hypercholesterolemic fat-fed rabbits. *Arteriosclerosis* 1987;7:9–23.
21. Rosenfeld ME, Tsukada T, Chait A, Bierman EL, Gown AM, Ross R. Fatty streak expansion and maturation in Watanabe heritable hyperlipemic and comparably hypercholesterolemic fat-fed rabbits. *Arteriosclerosis* 1987;7:24–34.

Atherosclerosis Reviews, Volume 21,
edited by A. Leaf and P. C. Weber.
Raven Press, Ltd., New York © 1990.

Hypertension:

The Coronary Heart Disease Dilemma

Paul Leren

*Department of Medicine, Oslo University Medical School, Ullevaal Hospital,
Medical Outpatient Clinic, 0407 Oslo 4, Norway*

Hypertension is a well-established risk factor for the development of coronary heart disease (CHD); however, the lowering of blood pressure by drugs has failed to give definite CHD protection. This is the hypertension–coronary dilemma, and a most embarrassing situation because CHD is a major health problem in most countries in the Western world. This is still true despite the fact that many countries have observed a marked reduction in the incidence of CHD. From 1970 to 1985 the U.S., Australia, Canada, and Japan experienced a reduction in CHD deaths of 49, 46, 41, and 39%, respectively, in men aged 30 to 69 years. The corresponding figures for women in the same age group are 48, 51, 43, and 53% (1).

In Europe, the CHD epidemiologic situation varies. In most of the traditionally high CHD countries, such as the Nordic countries, Northern Ireland and Scotland, a less pronounced decrease in the CHD mortality rate has been observed, averaging 11% (range: 3 to 23%). However, in many Eastern European countries CHD mortality is increasing at an alarming rate. From 1970 to 1985, the average CHD death rate in men, aged 30 to 69 years in Romania, Poland, Yugoslavia, Bulgaria, Hungary, the German Democratic Republic, and Czechoslovakia increased by an average of 48% (range: 10 to 90) (1).

The difference in CHD mortality between East and West Germany—9% decrease in West Germany and a 21% increase in East Germany (1)—is an interesting feature and a strong indication that there exists essential difference in living conditions between the two countries.

CAN CHD BE PREVENTED BY MODIFYING RISK FACTORS?

The main risk factors for developing CHD are hyperlipidemia, hypertension, and tobacco smoking. Isolated controlled smoking trials are most difficult to perform, and only one trial has been carried out, and without conclusive results (2).

Lipid Intervention

Adequately designed primary intervention studies have shown that the effects of a cholesterol-lowering diet alone cannot prevent CHD. In the Oslo Diet Heart Study (3,4), strict diet intervention in 412 postmyocardial infarction patients achieved a mean total cholesterol reduction of 17.6% versus 3.7% in the control group; the 5-year incidence of major coronary relapses was 61% versus 81% ($p = 0.05$).

The Oslo Study primary prevention trial was a two-factor study of high-risk, healthy men who smoked and had elevated cholesterol levels. At $8\frac{1}{2}$ years follow-up, the CHD incidence and total mortality was reduced by 42% ($p = 0.02$) and 36% ($p = 0.05$), respectively, as compared with the control group (5). However, the most convincing evidence has been obtained in monofactorial lipid intervention studies using lipid-lowering drugs.

The Lipid Research Clinics Coronary Primary Prevention Trial using cholestyramine (6), the WHO Drug Trial using clofibrate (7), the Coronary Drug Project using clofibrate and niacine (8), and the Helsinki Heart Study using gemfibrozil (9) all achieved positive effects on blood lipids and a reduced CHD incidence rate, but no significant reduction of total mortality. The Blanckenhorn Study using colestipol and niacine (10), and the NHLBI Study using cholestyramine (11) demonstrated an angiographically assessed decrease of the progression of coronary atherosclerosis as compared with untreated control groups.

Thus, it has been shown that CHD can be prevented by improving the lipid profile. Therefore, it is probable that adverse effects on blood lipids as caused by some antihypertensive drugs may have the opposite effects on CHD, diminishing or nullifying the beneficial effect of blood pressure reduction.

Hypertension Treatment

Through numerous epidemiologic studies, has been established that hypertension is a definite and important risk factor for the development of CHD even in countries where high-cholesterol levels are seen (such as most Western nations). This is in contrast to the epidemiologic situation in certain Eastern countries. In some of these countries where low-cholesterol levels are prevalent, CHD is extremely low despite a rather high prevalence of hypertension. It is probably so because hypertension needs the metabolic basis of a certain lipid level to become an atherogenic factor of clinical importance. In many countries this metabolic basis is endemic and hypertension is recognized as a definite CHD risk factor.

In the Multiple Risk Factor Intervention Trial (MRFIT) of about 350,000 men, aged 30 to 57 years (12), the 6-year CHD mortality gradient was 7.2 and 5.1, respectively, whether systolic blood pressure was ≥ 175 mm Hg or <115

mm Hg, and diastolic pressure was ≥115 mm Hg or <75 mm Hg. In the Oslo Study, a 12-year follow-up of 16,206 healthy men, aged 40 to 49 years (13), the fatal and nonfatal CHD incidence gradient was 2.6 and 3.6, respectively, whether systolic and diastolic pressure was in the first or fifth quintile of blood pressure distribution.

Despite this well-established association between hypertension and CHD, numerous hypertension drug trials have failed to provide a definite protection against CHD.

Recently published overview analyses of hypertension trials (14,15), including up to 43,000 patients and over 125,000 patients-years of observation conclude that a definite CHD protection has not been achieved. Such overview analysis of clinical trials can be criticized. However, also when looking at each trial separately, the conclusion of no definite benefit with regard to CHD holds true.

A special concern is the Hypertension Detection and Follow-up Program (HDFP) (16). In this study both randomized groups received drug treatment, one group more intensely (special care) than the other (referred care), and a difference in CHD incidence was observed in favor of the SC-group. Certainly, this is an indication of a beneficial effect of antihypertension drug therapy on CHD, but it is not proof. In his overview analysis of clinical trials in mild hypertension, Holme (14) presents odds ratios for all trials combined, with and without HDFP (stratum I). Inclusion of HDFP, changes the odds ratio from 0.97 (95% confidence limit 0.84–1.12) to 0.92 (0.82–1.03). Indications of even untoward effects on CHD from drug treatment of hypertension (diuretics and β-blockers) have been reported (17,18).

POSSIBLE REASONS FOR THE HYPERTENSION DRUG TREATMENT FAILURE IN CHD PROTECTION

In MRFIT (19), the 6-year CHD mortality gradient was 3.5 whether total serum cholesterol was ≥6.3 mmol/liter or ≤4.7 mmol/liter. In the 12-year follow-up of 16,206 men in Oslo Study (13), the incidence of fatal and nonfatal CHD was increased 5.7 times from a total cholesterol value in the first quintile as compared with the fifth quintile in the cholesterol distribution at screening. In that study it also was shown that total cholesterol is related positively to the degree of coronary-raised atherosclerotic lesions at autopsy, whereas HDL cholesterol was related strongly and inversely (20), and that there is an independent and significant negative association between the coronary death rate and premortal HDL cholesterol levels, whether the degree of coronary atherosclerosis is advanced, medium, or moderate (21).

The Framingham Study group (22) has estimated the relative CHD predictive power of various lipid fractions. From the follow-up results it is concluded that compared with total cholesterol, the CHD predictive power of LDL cholesterol and HDL cholesterol is more than 2 and 7 times, respectively, stronger. The strongest CHD predictive power, more than 8 times that of total cholesterol alone, was found to be associated with the ratio of HDL to total cholesterol. In the British Regional Heart Study (23), the superiority of HDL cholesterol over total cholesterol in predicting CHD was not confirmed, the two fractions showing about equal strength. Nevertheless, extensive epidemiologic studies and intervention trials have provided convincing evidence that blood lipids play a crucial role in the development of CHD.

ANTIHYPERTENSIVE DRUGS AND BLOOD LIPIDS

Based on two major reviews (24,25), the lipid profiles of the most commonly used antihypertensive drugs are as follows: Diuretics, nonselective and selective β-blockers have adverse effects on blood lipids, whereas β-blockers with strong intrinsic sympatomimetic activity are lipid neutral. Lipid neutral are also calcium-channel blockers, ACE inhibitors, labetalol, and methyldopa. α-Blockers have a favourable lipid profile.

The clinical importance of the observed metabolic effects of antihypertensive drugs is still uncertain, and caution should be exercised when it comes to practical implications. However, the fact that CHD has been shown to be preventable by modification of an adverse lipid profile, should lead to serious consideration of both the pressure lowering and the metabolic effects of antihypertensive drugs. Therapeutic changes in lifestyle are a critical component in the initial treatment of patients with hypertension. In patients with mild hypertension, the benefits derived from elimination of tobacco use, limitation of alcohol intake, weight loss, physical exercise, and, above all, dietary measures to reduce blood cholesterol, should be emphasized strongly. When nonpharmacologic measures alone are not satisfactory in controlling blood pressure, a strong argument can be made for the use of vasodilating agents as initial therapy.

First, drugs such as calcium-channel blockers, α-blockers, and ACE-inhibitors have a physiologically desirable way to lower blood pressure by decreasing increased peripheral vascular resistance, which is a hallmark of hypertension. Second, vasodilating drugs have no adverse effects on cardiac performance during physical activity. Third, these drugs exert no adverse effects on the most important causal factor for the development of CHD, the blood lipids.

CAN THE HYPERTENSION–CHD DILEMMA BE SOLVED?

It is not known whether the use of vasodilating drugs with their lipid neutrality or direct favourable lipid effects will prevent CHD when used in the treatment of hypertension. Only new trials with such drugs, adequately designed and controlled, can resolve this question. In the meantime there is a need for a reappraisal of conventional antihypertensive therapy, especially one that goes beyond the simple criterion of decreased blood pressure and takes into account all identified CHD-rich factors. Such considerations are valid for the primary prevention of CHD in "healthy" hypertensives who represent the vast majority of people receiving antihypertensive drugs today. The approach to hypertension treatment in patients already suffering from heart disease, e.g., heart failure, postmyocardial infarction with or without angina pectoris, is a different issue. Such patients are primarily in need of symptomatic treatment, in which the indication for the use of diuretics and β-adrenergic blockers are often mandatory.

In our efforts to prevent the, by far, most important complication of hypertension, that is, coronary heart disease, our hope at present is that vasodilating drugs can bring about a substantial reduction in CHD when used in hypertension treatment. Such drugs do have the potential to do so.

CONCLUSION

In the primary prevention of the prevailing complication of hypertension, i.e., coronary heart disease, there is a need for a reappraisal of conventional hypertension therapy, a therapy that goes beyond the simple criterion of decreased blood pressure and takes into account all identified coronary heart disease risk factors.

The vasodilating drugs, such as α-blockers, calcium-channel blockers, and ACE inhibitors with their physiologically correct mode of action and beneficial or neutral effects on lipid metabolism, do possess the potential to resolve the hypertension–CHD dilemma.

REFERENCES

1. Uemura K, Pisa Z. Trends in cardiovascular disease mortality in industrialized countries since 1950. *World Health STAT Q* 1988;41:155–178.
2. Rose G, Hamilton PJS. A randomised controlled trial of the effect on middle-aged men of advice to stop smoking. *Epidemiol Comm Health* 1978;32:275–281.
3. Leren P. The effect of plasma cholesterol lowering diet in male survivors of myocardial infarction. *Acta Med Scand* 1966;466(suppl):1–92.
4. Leren P. The Oslo diet heart study. Eleven-year report. *Circulation* 1970;42:935–942.
5. Hjermann I, Holme I, Leren P. Oslo Study diet and antismoking trial. Results after 102 months. *Am J Med* 1986;(suppl 2A):7–11.
6. Lipid Research Clinics Program. The lipid research clinics coronary primary prevention trial results. I Reduction in incidence of coronary heart disease. *JAMA* 1984;251:351–364.
7. WHO cooperative trial on primary prevention of ischemic heart disease using clofibrate to lower serum cholesterol: mortality follow-up. Report of the Committee of Principal Investigators. *Lancet* 1980;2:379–385.
8. Coronary Drug Project Research Group. Clofibrate and niacine in coronary artery disease. *JAMA* 1975;231:360–381.
9. Frick MH, Elo O, Haapa K, et al. Helsinki Heart Study. Primary prevention trial with gemfibrozil in middle-aged men with dyslipidemia. Safety of treatment, changes in risk factors, and incidence of coronary heart disease. *N Engl J Med* 1987;317:1237–1245.

10. Blankenhorn DH, Nessim SH, Johnson RI, et al. Beneficial effects of combined colestipol-niacine therapy on coronary atherosclerosis and coronary venous bypass grafts. *JAMA* 1987;257:3233–3240.

11. Levy RI, Brensike JF, Epstein SE, et al. The influence of changes in lipid values induced by cholestyramine and diet on progression of coronary artery disease: results of the NHLB I Type II coronary intervention study. *Circulation* 1984;69:325–337.

12. Stamler J, Neaton JD, Wenthon D. Blood pressure and risk of fatal coronary heart disease. *Hypertension* 1989;13(suppl 1):2–12.

13. Oslo Study. 12 year follow-up (in press).

14. Holme I. Drug treatment of mild hypertension to reduce the risk of CHD: Is it worth-while? *Stat Med* 1988;7:1109–1120.

15. MacMahon SW, Cutler JA, Neaton JD. Relationship of blood pressure to coronary and stroke morbidity and mortality in clinical trials and epidemiologic studies. *J Hypertens* 1986;4(suppl. 6):14–17.

16. Hypertension Detection and Follow-up Program Cooperative Group. Effect of stepped care on the incidence of myocardial infarction and angina pectoris. *Hypertension* 1984;6(suppl 1):198–206.

17. Leren P, Helgeland H. Coronary heart disease and treatment of hypertension. Some Oslo Study data. *Am J Med* 1986;80(suppl 2A):3–6.

18. Multiple Risk Factor Intervention Trial Research Group. Risk factor changes and mortality results. *JAMA* 1982;248:1465–1477.

19. Stamler J, Wentworth D, Neaton JD. Is relationship between serum cholesterol and risk of premature death from coronary heart disease continuous and graded? Finding in 356.222 primary screenees of the Multiple Risk Factor Intervention Trial (MRFIT). *JAMA* 1986;256:2823–2828.

20. Holme I, Enger SC, Helgeland A, et al. Risk factors and raised atherosclerosic lesions in coronary and cerebral arteries. Statistical analysis from the Oslo Study. *Arteriosclerosis* 1981;1:250–256.

21. Holme I, Solberg LA, Weissfeldt L, et al. Coronary risk factor and their pathway through coronary raised lesions, coronary stenoses and coronary death. Multivariate statistical analysis of an autopsy series: The Oslo Study. *Am J Cardiol* 1985;55:40–47.

22. Castelli WP, Anderson K. A population at risk. Prevalence of high cholesterol levels in hypertensive patients in the Framingham Study. *Am J Med* 1986;80(suppl. 2A):23–36.

23. Pocock SJ, Shaper AG, Phillips AN. Concentration of high density lipoprotein cholesterol, triglycerides, and total cholesterol in ischaemic heart disease. *Br Med J* 1989;298:998–1002.

24. Leren P. Effects of antihypertensive drugs on lipid metabolism. *Clin Ther* 1987;9:326–332.

25. Krone W, Naegele H. Effects of antihypertensives on plasma lipids and lipoprotein metabolism. *Am Heart J* 1988;116:1729–1734.

Atherosclerosis Reviews, Volume 21,
edited by A. Leaf and P. C. Weber.
Raven Press, Ltd., New York © 1990.

Antiatherosclerotic Potential of Calcium Antagonists

Fritz R. Bühler, *Paul Leren, †Paul R. Lichtlen,
‡Rodolfo Paoletti, and §Russell Ross

*Department of Research, University Hospital, Basel, Switzerland; *Department of
Medicine, Oslo University Medical School, Oslo, Norway; †Division of Cardiology,
Hannover Medical School, Hannover, F.R.G.; ‡Institute of Pharmacology and
Pharmacognosy, University of Milan, Milan, Italy; and §Department
of Pathology, University of Washington, Seattle, Washington*

Calcium antagonists have become cornerstones of antianginal and antihypertensive treatment in the last 25 years. The question now is whether calcium antagonists have additional cardioprotective effects. At an international workshop on atherosclerosis and its prevention and noninvasive therapy, the following issues were addressed during a roundtable discussion: (a) Is there evidence that calcium antagonists may affect the progression of atherosclerosis? (b) How do calcium antagonists interfere with other cardiovascular risk factors? (c) What are the possible mechanisms of the calcium antagonists' intervention with atherosclerosis development?

Based on findings of a parallel increase of arterial cholesterol and calcium vascular contents, an association between a derangement of calcium homeostasis and development of atherosclerosis has long been suspected (1). This concept has been revived by Fleckenstein, who demonstrated a 100-fold increase of calcium in aortic walls of elderly subjects as compared to young subjects (2). In cholesterol-fed rabbits, a fivefold increase in intracellular calcium concentration has been accounted for by increased plasma membrane calcium permeability in aortic smooth muscle cells (3). Although these findings do not prove a causal role of calcium, they do indicate the possibility that cellular calcium and thereby slow calcium-channel influx inhibition may influence the multiple mechanisms eventually leading to the development of the atherosclerotic lesion with its detrimental consequences.

EVIDENCE FOR ANTIATHEROSCLEROTIC EFFECTS OF CALCIUM ANTAGONISTS

Models have been developed—mainly cholesterol feeding of animals and tissue cultures of animal and human arterial cells—to facilitate the study of potential therapeutic interventions. There is ample support for all three types of calcium antagonists to blunt or prevent atherosclerotic lesions (4–6), but it remains to be shown to what extent this experience can be translated into clinical practice.

To date, there are two major clinical studies in keeping with the notion that calcium antagonists may reduce the development of atherosclerotic lesions or interfere with pre-existing narrowing of coronary arteries. In a very recent publication, Drs. Loaldi and Guazzi (7) showed a significantly lower number of new lesions and progression of pre-existing stenoses. Dr. Lichtlen expanded on his presentation of the International Nifedipine Trial on Anti-atherosclerotic Therapy Study at the meeting in Key West, Florida. Nifedipine was shown to reduce significantly the development of new lesions in patients with coronary artery bypass, though no effect was discernible on pre-existing lesions. It was pointed out that, in contrast to most animal studies, these effects were obtained with relatively low doses of nifedipine.

Dr. Ross raised the challenging question of why no regression of atherosclerotic lesions has been observed during nifedipine therapy. Here we are concerned with breakdown of connective tissue, removal of cellular elements as well as lipids, lipoproteins and lipoprotein breakdown products, and very little is known about the chronology of these regression processes. Although the necessity of calcium influx through the calcium channel was questioned by Dr. Thomas, its pivotal role is evident from antiatherosclerotic effects observed with a low-dose calcium antagonist regimen (8) and with calcium antagonists with largely different chemical structures but common slow calcium-channel entry–inhibiting properties (9). However, Dr. Paoletti emphasized the degree to which calcium antagonists penetrate into liposomal compartments inside the cell, which helps explain why some calcium antagonists may be more antiatherogenetic than others. Dr. Bühler mentioned the effects of other cardiovascular drugs that reduce vascular smooth muscle cell proliferation; these include the potassium channel opener minoxidil, the α_1-adrenoceptor blocker prazosin, and some of the β-blockers. He postulated the essential role of a reduction in cytosolic free calcium concentration, a common feature of all these agents.

POSSIBLE ANTIATHEROSCLEROTIC MECHANISMS

In addition to their well-documented prevention of cellular calcium overload, calcium antagonists seem to have beneficial effects on endothelial damage and perivascular inflammation. Thus, calcium antagonists may preserve endothelial-dependent vascular relaxation in cholesterol-fed rabbits (9), and this may be particularly relevant in light of endothelial derangements playing a key role in the development of atherosclerosis.

According to Dr. Ross, the invasion of smooth muscle cells from the media into the intima and their subsequent proliferation is one of the hallmarks of early plaque development. The smooth muscle cell in this process undergoes a modulation from contractile to synthetic phenotype, with subsequent proliferation and secretion of extracellular matrix components. Platelet-derived growth factor (PDGF) may be of major importance in this process (10), and it is of interest that the initial response to PDGF *in vitro* includes an elevation of intracellular free calcium concentration (11). For example, nifedipine retards the differentiation of contractile into synthetic smooth muscle cells in micromolar concentrations and inhibited DNA synthesis in cultured vascular smooth muscle cells, a feature less pronounced with verapamil and diltiazem. The relatively weak calcium antagonist flunarizin reduces plaque formation in electrically stimulated arteries of cholesterol-fed rabbits (12). Calcium antagonists have also been shown to inhibit migration of smooth muscle cells at very low concentrations. All of these findings can help to explain the beneficial effects of calcium antagonists during the early phase of plaque development. The common denominator for the actions of these different agents on smooth muscle cell proliferation remains to be defined.

The role of macrophages needs to be elucidated; they too seem to be affected by calcium antagonists. Dr. Paoletti mentioned that lipid loading or low-density lipoprotein (LDL)-receptor stimulation on macrophages can be blunted by calcium antagonists.

Dr. Ross focused on the role of overexposed macrophages and mural thrombi and the role in advanced lesions. More information is needed on the role of different cells involved (i.e., platelets, macrophages, endothelial, and vascular smooth muscle cells) with regard to cholesterol esterification or cholesterol ester hydrolysis, using concentrations of calcium antagonists close to those obtained during pharmacotherapy. It will be equally important to apply information obtained from rat or monkey tissue to human tissue.

INTERFERENCE WITH OTHER CARDIOVASCULAR RISK FACTORS

Overall, calcium antagonists have neutral, and in some studies even beneficial, effects on the plasma lipoprotein profile. Thus, in cholesterol-fed rabbits different calcium antagonists tended to decrease LDL-cholesterol and increase high-density lipoprotein (HDL)-cholesterol, but these effects are not necessarily linked to the antiatherosclerotic effect of calcium antagonists (13). Dr. Leren stated that in pharmacotherapy, calcium antagonists can be regarded as metabolically neutral.

Dr. Paoletti pointed to the evidence that calcium antagonists can influence the cellular metabolism of lipoproteins. Cholesterol is presented to the cells as LDL by binding to a specific cell surface receptor and subsequent internalization by pinocytosis. After delivery to lysosomes, cholesterol esters are hydrolyzed by lysosomal acid cholesterol esterase. In humans, reduction or congenital deficiency of acid cholesterol esterase leads to severe atherosclerosis, indicating the importance of this degradation pathway. Verapamil enhances binding and internalization of LDL in cultured human monocyte–derived macrophages, and the synthesis rate of LDL receptors in human fibroblasts increases with diltiazem and verapamil. This raises the possibility that calcium antagonists increase receptor-mediated lipoprotein clearance. Because fibroblasts do not seem to have voltage-sensitive slow calcium channels, these effects are likely to be caused by an action unrelated to the calcium channel–blocking activity of these compounds. In addition, decreased cholesterol ester deposition in macrophages has been observed with calcium antagonists, i.e., nifedipine, as well as the weak calcium agonist Bay K 8644. In rabbit smooth muscle cells, lysosomal cholesterol esterase was doubled by nifedipine without effect on cytoplasmic cholesterol esterase (14).

Glucose intolerance and insulin resistance factors were discussed by Dr. Bühler. Both the angiotensin-converting enzyme inhibitor captopril and the α_1-blocker prazosin have been shown to improve insulin resistance and, thereby, glucose tolerance (15). In the case of calcium antagonists, however, the picture is unclear. As Dr. Paoletti pointed out, calcium antagonists stimulate *de novo* synthesis of insulin receptors, and it may well turn out that calcium antagonists beneficially affect insulin resistance. Drs. Leaf and Weber (the meeting organizers) raised the issue that aspirin, for example, deals at the level of vascular lesions yet does not interfere with the above mechanisms.

Smoking may be another confounding factor. Dr. Lichtlen outlined the effects of nifedipine on new lesion development and clarified equal benefit in smokers and nonsmokers.

The antihypertensive efficacy of all types of calcium antagonists is now well established (16), and many studies have shown that they also reduce left ventricular hypertrophy—which is regarded as another risk factor.

PREVENTION OF REINFARCTION?

Unlike the overall benefit of β-blockers in secondary prevention, the result of a recent meta-analysis showed that, in general, calcium antagonists do not reduce reinfarctional mortality following sustained myocardial infarction (17). There was even an indication of higher mortality owing to increased sudden death rates during postinfarct therapy with calcium antagonists (despite the fact that over one-third of the patients were receiving a β-blocker as well). However, meta-analysis may not tell the full story. There is no indication that the preventive effect seen with β-blockers in Q-wave infarct would hold true in non-Q-wave infarctions. It is conceivable that in this abortive form of myocardial infarction, calcium antagonists find their cardioprotective place. In fact, diltiazem has been shown—against a strong background of β-blockers—to prevent rein-farction and mortality in patients who survived a non-Q-wave infarction. To date, only diltiazem has been so precisely analyzed. Similar breakdowns of re-sults from studies with verapamil and dihydropyridines are still awaited. The Danish Verapamil Infarction Trial II may provide fresh and positive infor-mation.

There is considerable evidence that calcium antagonists influence important mechanisms involved in the atherosclerotic disease process and that they are effective in many animal models of atherosclerosis. In current literature, there is little to suggest an antiatherosclerotic effect of these drugs in humans. Calcium antagonists interfere with almost any process involved in atherosclerotic lesion development, but appropriate trials to test this hypothesis have yet to be per-formed in humans.

REFERENCES

1. Bürger M. Die chemischen Altersveränderungen an Gefässen. *Z Neurol Psychiatr* 1939;167: 273–280.
2. Fleckenstein A, Frey M, von Witzleben H. Vascular calcium overload—a pathogenetic factor in arteriosclerosis and its neutralization by calcium antagonists. In: Kaltenbach M, Neufeld HN, eds. *Proceedings of the 6th international Adalat symposium. New therapy of ischemic heart disease and hypertension*. Amsterdam: Excerpta Medica, 1983:36–52.
3. Strickberger SA, Russek LN, Phair RD. Evidence for increased aortic plasma membrane cal-cium transport caused by experimental atherosclerosis in rabbits. *Circ Res* 1988;62:75–80.
4. Weinstein DB, Heider JG. Antiatherogenic properties of calcium antagonists. *Am J Cardiol* 1987;59:163B–172B.
5. Henry PD, Bentley KL. Suppression of atherogenesis in cholesterol-fed rabbits treated with nifedipine. *J Clin Invest* 1981;68:1366–1369.
6. Fleckenstein A, Frey M, Zorn H, Fleckenstein-Grün G. Calcium, a neglected key factor in hypertension and arteriosclerosis: experimental vasoprotection with calcium antagonists or ACE inhibitors. In: Laragh DH, Brenner BM, eds. *Hypertension: pathophysiology–diagnosis and management*. New York: Raven Press, 1990:471–509.
7. Loaldi A, Polese A, Montorsi P, et al. Comparison of nifedipine, propanolol and isosorbide dinitrate on angiographic progression and regression of coronary arterial narrowings in angina pectoris. *Am J Cardiol* 1989;64:433–439.
8. Habib JB, Bossaller C, Wells S, Williams C, Morisett JD, Henry PD. Preservation of endotheli-um-dependent vascular relaxation in cholesterol-fed rabbits by treatment with the calcium blocker PN 2001 10. *Circ Res* 1986;58:305–309.
9. Kazda S, Grunt M, Hirth C, Preis W, Stasch J-P. Calcium antagonism and protection of tissue from calcium damage. *J Hypertens* 1987;5(suppl 4):37–42.
10. Ross R, Glomset J. The pathogenesis of atherosclerosis. *N Engl J Med* 1976;295:420–425.
11. Moolenaar WH, Tertoolen LGJ, de Laat SW. Growth factors immediately raise cytoplasmic free calcium in human fibroblasts. *J Biol Chem* 1984;259:8066–8072.
12. Betz E, Hämmerle H, Strohschneider T. Inhibitory actions of calcium entry blockers on experi-mental atheromas. In: Godfraind T, ed. *Calcium entry blockers and tissue protection*. New York: Raven Press, 1985,117–128.
13. Blumlein SL, Sievers R, Kidd P, Parmley WW. Mechanism of protection from atherosclerosis by verapamil in the cholesterol-fed rabbit. *Am J Cardiol* 1984;54:884–889.
14. Etingin OR, Hajjar DP. Nifedipine increases cholesterol ester hydrolytic activity in lipid-laden smooth muscle cells. *J Clin Invest* 1985;75:1554–1558.

15. Pollare T, Lithell H, Berne C. A comparison of the effects of hydrochlorothiazide and captopril on glucose and lipid metabolism in patients with hypertension. *N Engl J Med* 1989;321:868–873.
16. Bühler FR. Calcium antagonists for antihypertensive care. In: Bühler FR, Laragh JH, eds. *Handbook of hypertension, vol. 13.* Amsterdam: Elsevier, 1990 (in press).
17. Held PH, Yusuf S, Furberg CD. Calcium channel blockers in acute myocardial infarction and unstable angina: an overview. *Br Med J* 1989;299:1187–1192.